Psychology for Nurses

PSYCHOLOGY FOR NURSES

SWATI SHARMA
MA (Psychology)

UNIVERSITY SCIENCE PRESS
(An Imprint of Laxmi Publications Pvt. Ltd.)

BENGALURU • CHENNAI • COCHIN • GUWAHATI • HYDERABAD
JALANDHAR • KOLKATA • LUCKNOW • MUMBAI • RANCHI • NEW DELHI
INDIA • USA • GHANA • KENYA

PSYCHOLOGY FOR NURSES

Printed and bound in India
Typeset at Shubham Composer, Delhi
First Edition : 2015
ISBN 978-93-83828-62-3

Branches

✆	Bengaluru	080-26 75 69 30	
✆	Chennai	044-24 34 47 26,	24 35 95 07
✆	Cochin	0484-237 70 04,	405 13 03
✆	Guwahati	0361-254 36 69,	251 38 81
✆	Hyderabad	040-27 55 53 83,	27 55 53 93
✆	Jalandhar	0181-222 12 72	
✆	Kolkata	033-22 27 43 84	
✆	Lucknow	0522-220 99 16	
✆	Mumbai	022-24 91 54 15,	24 92 78 69
✆	Ranchi	0651-220 44 64	

PUBLISHED IN INDIA BY

UNIVERSITY SCIENCE PRESS
(An Imprint of Laxmi Publications Pvt.Ltd.)

An ISO 9001:2008 Certified Company
113, GOLDEN HOUSE, DARYAGANJ,
NEW DELHI - 110002, INDIA
Telephone : 91-11-4353 2500, 4353 2501
Fax : 91-11-2325 2572, 4353 2528
www.laxmipublications.com info@laxmipublications.com

C—
Printed at : Repro Knowledgecast Limited, Thane

Dedication

This book is dedicated

to my father

PREFACE

Psychology for Nurses is a book for nursing students across India and SAARC nations. This is a textbook based on the syllabus outlined by Indian Nursing Council. Syllabi from various universities across India were reviewed and contents of the book were designed accordingly. This book not only throws light on theoretical issues but also on practicum's attached with the theory.

Psychology for Nurses will be successful where just theory is taught and also in colleges where practicals are also conducted. Only precise and important concepts are included so that the students' curiosity and interest remain entwined while they read.

I wish best of luck to my readers and hope that it will be successful in the Nursing field.

Suggestions for the improvement of the book in the forthcoming edition will be gratefully acknowledged. Please do feel free to share your views with me at swati9948@yahoo.com

—Author

CONTENTS

SECTION-II: PRACTICAL

SECTION-I

Theory

1

INTRODUCTION TO PSYCHOLOGY

TOPICS COVERED IN THIS CHAPTER

- History and Origin of Science of Psychology
- Schools of Psychology
- Psychology as a Science
- Methods in Psychology
- Techniques Employed in Psychology
- Major Fields of Psychology

HISTORY AND ORIGIN OF SCIENCE OF PSYCHOLOGY

Radha describes herself as cool and happy. Now as a psychology student how would you describe cool and happy. Is it because she has got a smile on her face, looks relaxed as she is seated as being stuffed inside a gunny bag. Is it you would say that parasympathetic nervous system makes her relaxed or she is happy because she appraises the situation or event around her to be exciting. Is it the cognitions, physiology or interaction of both mind and body describes her as happy and cool. Let's begin with the roots from where psychology was born.

Psychology originated from philosophy. But the split from philosophy as a separate field of study was a little over 100 years ago. Psychology in the broad sense, means the science of mind because 'psyche' means self/soul and 'logos' denotes a reasoned account. Like physics, chemistry and often natural sciences, psychology too seeks to discover some general principles or laws. Natural sciences investigate the nature of physical phenomena and try to formulate a law or laws governing the phenomena. Psychology on the contrary, investigates the psychical or mental phenomena which is also natural. There are different viewpoints that try to define psychology. In the history of psychology, there are deep differences of opinion about what psychology should study and how it should study. This was represented by different schools of psychology.

Descartes (1596–1650) the reputed French philosopher is called the 'father of modem philosophy'. His interest was in the knowledge of 'self' which lead to the analysis of consciousness. Thus, the problem of psychology arose. He said soul, body, consciousness and nervous system are separate but interact with each other. If we study the various definitions of psychology, they changed over a period of time, we would get an idea of the subject matter and nature of psychology. It would also lead to a brief history of development of psychology as a science.

In the history of western psychology Aristotle (384–322 BC) is said to be the father of psychology as he was of many other sciences like logic, politics, etc., according to him the subject matter of psychology was the soul which he defined as an entity which realizes an idea. The science of soul was philosopher's definition which was upheld upto nineteenth century. Owing to the difficulty that by such a definition psychology became identified with metaphysics, the traditional psychology of the 19th century modified the definition and called itself, the science of mind. Mind has two aspects a as it appears to us through behaviour and as the reality behind the phenomenal mind.

Another definition acceptable during the last century was 'psychology is the science of consciousness—consciousness is the seat of mind. Thus, concept of mind as consciousness was received from Descartes.

All other definitions given at that time were: J. Dewey: psychology is the science of facts or phenomena of self. Wundt defined it as the science of experience by experience he meant immediate experience. Watson says that psychology is that division of natural science which takes human behaviour-the doing and sayings both learned and unlearned, of people as subject matter'. Thus for Watson 'psychology is a purely objective, experimental branch of natural science. Mc Dougall defined psychology as the positive science of conduct or behaviour. He modified it many years later, it the science which aims to give us better understanding and control of the behaviour of the organism as a whole. According to R. S. Woodworth, psychology is the science of the activities of the individual mental activities-he explained are grouped under knowing, feeling and doing. Koffka said that, psychology is the scientific study of the behaviour of living creatures in their context with the outer world. Boring says that it is the study of human nature—the study of man, man as a living being, acting in an ever changing world, responding to things and events and other people.

Some modern viewpoints are: Garderner Murphy, it is the science that studies the responses which living individuals make to their environment. Kagan and Havemann, psychology is the science that systematically studies and attempt to explain observable behaviour and its relationships to the unseen mental processes that go on inside the organism and to external events in the environment. Morgan and King, psychology is the science of human and animal behaviour it includes the application of this science to human problems. R. Baron, psychology is the science of behaviour and cognitive processes.

SCHOOLS OF PSYCHOLOGY

Structuralism

This early school of thought grew up around the ideas of Wilhelm Wundt and Edward B. Titchener. According to them, the mind is composed of the basic units: sensation, ideas, image and emotion. It is also referred to as content psychology. The method used by structuralists to discover these basic units of mind was introspection. Subjects were trained to report as objectively as possible what they experienced in connection with a certain stimulus, disregarding the meanings they had come to associate with the stimulus. For example: what is blue? shortcoming of this school was that it could not explain how these elements of consciousness or mind functions. Introspection involved a lot of subjectivity. Structure of mind could not be observed.

Functionalism

It emerged where John Dewey and James Angell and Harvey Carr proposed that psychology should study "what mind and behaviour do". William James was interested in studying how the mind functions (worked) so that an organism could adapt to its environment and helps in its survival. Functionalists were influenced by Darwin's views on survival for the fittest. Functionalists did experiments on the ways in which learning, memory, problem solving and motivation help people and animals to adapt to their environment.

Behaviourism

This school of thought was given by John B. Watson. He restricted to the study of behaviour—the observable activities of people and animals. He emphasized that data of psychology should be observable and measurable. There was emphasis on learned rather than unlearned behaviour. It denied the emphasis on innate behaviour as he did not believe. There was emphasis on conditioned response. Its elements were conditioned responses rather than sensations, images or emotions. Its focus was on animal behaviour. Watson believed that there are no differences between animal and human behaviour *i.e.,* we can learn much about our own behaviour what animals do. It rejected introspection and emphasized upon objectivity.

Gestalt Psychology

It was founded in Germany. Gestalt means "form" or configuration. Gestalt psychologists believed that mind is best understood in terms of the ways elements are organized. For example: When you look at the dots your mental experience is not just dots but of square and triangle sitting on a line. It is a organisation of the dots and their relationship that determine the mental experience you have. Gestalt psychologists in their opposition to structuralism was that mental experience depends on the patterning and organization of elements and is not due to compounding of elements.

Psychoanalysis

It is not a school of psychology but has had a great impact on the thinking and theorizing of many psychologists. Psychoanalysis was introduced by Sigmund Freud. Freud developed a theory of behaviour and mind which said that much of what we do and think results from urges or drives, which seek expression in behaviour and thought, in way like dreams, slips of speech and unconscious mannerisms. These urges are hidden *i.e.,* they are unconscious and the expression of these is unconscious motivation.

Modern Perspectives

In the last 50 years, psychologists give a variety of viewpoints which describe and understand behaviour. These are:

Neurobiological perspective

This approach studies the activity in our brains and other parts of the nervous system, hormones released by our glands and other bodily changes induce such processes which are intimately linked to everything we do, think, feel or say. It explain: what happens inside our body when we think, listen to music, grow hungry or sexually aroused (all psychological events) are represented in some manner by activity of brain and nervous system. For example: perception can be studied by recording the activity of nerve cells in the brain as the eye is exposed to various visual displays. Because of complexity of brain and human brains are seldom available for study, tremendous gaps exists in knowledge of neural functioning.

Cognitive approach

It focuses on thinking, memory and decision making, perception and language. Cognition refers "To the mental processes of perception, memory and information processing by which individual acquires knowledge, solves problems and plans for the future." Cognitive psychology is the scientific study of cognition. Its goal is to conduct experiments and develop theories that how mental processes are organized and function. But to know how mental processes function, neurobiological explanations are needed. Kenneth Craik, cognitive psychologist proposed that brain is like a computer or an "information processing system". Incoming information selected, compared and combined with other information already in memory, transformed, rearranged and so on. The response output depends on these internal processes and the state at the moment. Protocol analysis (updated version of introspection) here the subject thinks out aloud and provides verbal reports of his or mental activities while performing a task.

Evolutionary Perspective

It is an approach which studies the adaptive problem humans have faced over the course of evolution and the behavioural mechanism that have evolved in response to environmental pressures.

Modern psychologists believe that like other species on our planet, human beings have an evolutionary history which equips them with inherited tendencies or dispositions.

Sociocultural Perspective

According to this perspective, an individual's perception, thinking, feelings and actions are strongly influenced by the social and cultural systems in which they live.

Multicultural Perspective

Ethnic and cultural diversity has increased greatly during recent decades in many countries around the world and the multicultural perspective studies all aspects of behaviour which are strongly influenced by factors related to cultural and ethnic identity.

PSYCHOLOGY AS A SCIENCE

A science is a body of systematized knowledge that is gathered by carefully observing and measurements. Psychologists do experiments and make observations which others can repeat. The apparatus used have several characteristics. These are:

- It measures accurately and consistently within the range where the stimulus or response is produced.

- It should not itself produce any effect that would obscure or alter the event being investigated.
- It should provide a means of collecting automatically.
- Psychological tests such as paper and pencil tests to assess intelligence. Where the subject's intelligence is the antecedent, his intelligence quotient is the consequence. The standardized procedure of administering the test is the means of controlling the situation.

They obtain data often in the form of quantitative measurements, which often can verify. This scientific approach is very different from forming opinions on the basis of individuals experiences or arguing from premises that no one can test. Thus experiments and observations are at the core of scientific psychology. Systematic study : as a science psychology is systematic data from experiment and observation are essential, but for this to make some sense in helping us understand events they must be organized in some way. Scientific theories are important tools for the organization of observed facts. To some people the word theory simply means someone's unsupported and unfounded opinion/notion of how things ought to be done or a set of abstract principles that do not work in practical situations. However, in science, theories are general principles which summarize many observations and predict what can be expected to happen in the new situations. As new data are obtained, theories are subject to modifications or scrapped in favour of new ones which do a better job of summarizing and predicting.

Measurement: It is defined as the assignment of numbers to objects or events according to certain rules. In physical scales, it is in terms of length, time, temperature, etc. Measurement in psychology is often more difficult because: what are the yardsticks of happiness or friendship for example. Psychologists have devised many ingenious tests to assign numbers to them. Experiments are often designed to arrange observations in such a way as to use physical measures of space and time to tell us about psychological events. For example, we can count the number of times a person behaves one way in one situation and another way in another situation or we measure the time taken to make a response in one situation or another.

METHODS OF PSYCHOLOGY

Experimental Method

It is the most precise, planned and controlled observation. Experiment is the most scientific research method. Because it only make possible controlled observations, variation of factors, perfect quantifications, rigorous, objective checking of hypothesis and observations can be repeated. The main weakness of the experiment are that an experiment is an artificial situation. The experimental data obtained under artificial situation may not reveal natural and actual working of mental processes as under normal conditions. As, Thorndike's experimental animals had no choice but to exhibit trial and error learning. If an organism is enclosed in a maze with high walls which would prevent him from any insight or oversight, he would be forced to try and error. Further, human behaviour is complex and what is observed in just one experimental situation may be inadequate. Behaviour is extremely variable. Moreover, no two individuals are alike so results or findings cannot be always generalized. A physicist can duplicate the conditions of his experiments like temperature and pressure. But psychologist cannot keep the amount of experience same of the subject. According to G.S. Klein, the appearance of significant relations was often prevented by the rigourous experiment procedure of keeping variables constant. Experiments cannot handle the patterns of covert or overt behaviour, violent types of action as they do not fit the lab setting. Nor can experimenter test the entire gamut of human drives and feelings. It is so because experimentalist studies but a part of human behaviour but he studies it with great precision. The clinician studies the totality of human behaviour.

Observation

Observation involves looking and listening to what other people say or behave. There are many types of observation methods. Participant observation is a qualitative method with roots in traditional ethnographic research. Participant observation or field observation is one of the most demanding and common methods of qualitative data collection method. It requires the researcher to become a participant in the specific culture or context under study. Participant observation often requires months or years of intensive work because the researcher needs to become accepted as a natural part of the culture in order to assure that the observations are part of natural phenomenon.

Laboratory observation or non-participant observation is different in a number of ways. First, the non participant observer doesn't typically try to become a participant in the culture under study the researcher is watching rather than taking part. Technology can be a useful part of direct observation or non participant observation. For instance, one can videotape the phenomenon or observer from behind. Here the observer is not bias about his observations. Second, is non-participant observer tends to be more focused than participant observation. Here, the researcher manipulates the independent variable under study. The field observer takes his observations in a natural setting. Non-participant observer is taking the observation in an artificial setting. Another disadvantage of participant observation is the difficulty of documenting the data—it is hard to write down everything that is important while you are in the act of participating and observing. The non-participant observation tends not to take as long as participant observation. It is so because the laboratory conditions are set where the independent variable is manipulated by the experimenter. So cannot be continued to for long as experimental conditions are not met for such durations. Finally, in field observation it requires conscious effort at objectivity because method is inherently subjective.

The Case Study Method

The method has been adopted from the medical sciences. An attempt is made to go through the history of an individual from the period of infancy onwards. This is done with the view to assess the various factors, heredity and environmental that helped in developing the individuals personality. The method is often used in studying of normal behaviour. The main objective is to detect and diagnose specific problems and suggest therapeutic measures to rehabilitate the individual in his environment. The information is obtained through observation, interview, questionnaires. A case study is an in-depth study of one person or an organization. The next form of research that psychologists frequently use in their work is called a case study. Unlike a survey, a case study closely studies one individual as opposed to a group of individuals. Case studies can be compared and contrasted to help further analyze data.

Survey Method

This method involves asking large number of individuals to complete questionnaire designed to yield information on specific aspect of their behaviour or attitudes. Surveys are often repeated over long periods of time in order to track down shifts in public opinions or actual behaviour. The method offers some real advantages.

(a) Large amount of information can be gathered with relative case

(b) Shifts over time can be readily noted.

Limitations:

(a) People may fail to respond accurately or truthfully.

(b) The results of surveys are useful only if the person questioned are truly representative of large groups to whom the findings are to be generalized.

TECHNIQUES EMPLOYED IN PSYCHOLOGY

Psychological Tests

Psychological tests are designed to measure intelligence, personality, feelings, motives, attitudes etc. They are set of questions designed scientifically and arranged systematically which could be answered verbally or by using hands, fingers, etc; they help in exploring behaviour and comparative studies.

Interview

It is a verbal technique for obtaining data. It is a face to face interaction. It has a goal to achieve — understanding an individual —the personality dimension. Young defined it as "a systematic method by which a person enters more or less imaginatively into the life of a comparative stranger." Interview schedule is a tool of social sciences. It involves a set of questions related to social, political and cognitive issues. It is a tool to get information from the respondent concerning various psychological and sociological issues. Interview means, "conversation with a purpose" by Bingham and Moore, 1941.

Questionnaires

According to Bogardus, "a questionnaire is a list of questions given to a respondent to answer. It secures standardized results that can be tabulated and treated statistically." They are prepared with the specific purpose of assessing one or more psychological characteristic of the individual. They are generally standardized so that they measure what they supposed to and would provide authentic, dependable and consistent results within the units of their applicability. They can be used on an individual or on a group.

MAJOR FIELDS OF PSYCHOLOGY

General Psychology

Explains basic principles of general processes—learning, perception, memory, thinking, motivation, etc.

Physiological Psychology

Tries to study the fundamental causes of behaviour.

Comparative Psychology

Studies animal and human behaviour.

School and Educational Psychology

Concerned with increasing efficiency of learning in school by applying their psychological knowledge about learning and motivation. Diagnosing learning difficulties and trying to remedy them.

Developmental Psychology

Developmental psychologists try to understand the complex behaviour by studying their beginnings, and the orderly ways in which they change with time. Since changes in behaviour occur rapidly in early years of life, child psychology, the study of children behaviour comprises a large part of developmental psychology. The changes also occur in adolescence, adulthood and old age and so study of these changes also a part of development psychology.

Industrial and Organizational Psychology

The first application of psychology to the problem of industries and organization was the use of intelligence and aptitude tests in selecting employees. The problem of management employees training, supervision, improving communication within the organization, counseling employees. Psychological principles are applied to practical problems of work and commerce.

Social Psychology

It includes the study of the ways in which we perceive other people and how those perceptions affect on behaviour towards them. It involves concerted efforts to understand the determinants of interpersonal influences and of attitude change. Prejudices stereotypes -their affect on interaction.

Abnormal and Clinical Psychology

Diagnosis of psychological disorders and their treatment by means of psychotherapy.

REFLECT YOURSELF

1. Discuss psychology as a science.
2. What is the scope of psychology?
3. What are the research methods used in psychology?

2

BIOLOGY OF BEHAVIOUR

TOPICS COVERED IN THIS CHAPTER

- Introduction
- Neuron and Synapse
- Neurotransmitter
- Nervous System
- Brain
- Glandular Controls of Behaviour
- Functions of Various Glands
- Muscular Controls of Behaviour

INTRODUCTION

Our daily life is filled with examples that show the pivotal role played by our brain in behaviour. This chapter talks about biology of behaviour. Biology of behaviour means physiological bases of behaviour. It is physiological because it predicts behaviour by using knowledge of how the organs and systems of the body work. Our behaviour is generally guided by role of neurotransmitters released by neurons in the synaptic cleft supported by integrated systems of central nervous system and peripheral nervous system. These structural relationships between muscular and glandular controls determine behaviour in similar situations or different circumstances.

Body and Mind Relationship

Behaviour that is elicited by a stimulus is known as a response. Behaviour has cognitive, affective and conative components. The process or result of the unification of these components into a whole is called integrated response.

Psychology studies the relationship between mind and body. Mind and body affect each other. The mind operates at the levels of thinking, emotion and action. Mind and body cannot act independently on parallel lines. This is meant by integrated response *i.e.,* inseparable from each other.

When angry thoughts cross your brain, they stimulate both the halves of the autonomic nervous system—the sympathetic which energizes you and the parasympathetic which calms you down. You may consider the former as a car's accelerator and the latter as a brake.

Action of mind upon body

All physical and motor activities begin by the motivation in the mind. Negative emotions like fear, anger and jealousy produce illness. They make us depressed. Emotional conflicts lie at the root of peptic ulcers, coronary heart diseases, blood pressure and neurosis.

Deep thinking and concentration can cause physical fatigue. Soldiers win the war by putting extra effort when their morale is high.

Action of body upon mind

Rise in blood pressure leads to mental excitement. Fatigue retards intellectual activity. Sudden emotion causes mental imbalance. Constipation makes irritable. Hyperthyroidism leads to excitement and hypothyroidism causes lethargy. Bad throat can reduce concentration.

Heredity and Environment

Heredity refers to the biological process of transmission of certain biological and psychological characteristics from parents to their children through genes.

Studies by **Galton** and others into the ancestral history of twins, scientists, kings, judges and artists clearly demonstrated that distinctive mental ability is the result of inheritance rather than education.

Many aspects of human behaviour and development ranging from physical characteristics such as height, weight, eye and skin colour, the complex patterns of social and intellectual behaviour are influenced by a person's genetic endowment. It also includes physical deficiencies and the nature of glandular functioning.

Functional units of heredity are genes. Heredity is source of both similarities and differences among individuals. Biological inheritance is determined by chromosomes and genes. Females have 23 pairs of XX chromosomes. Males have 22 pairs of XX plus two singles represented as X and Y. The X and Y are called sex chromosomes because sex depends upon XX and XY combinations. The heredity factors hidden within the chromosomes are the genes. They are the packet of chemicals strung along the chromosomes like small beads on a thread. Within each chromosome there are about 1000 genes. These genes contain two chemical substances DNA and RNA which are responsible for transmitting the genetic code message from parent to offspring.

A form of mental retardation is due to the presence of an extra chromosome instead of two in the twenty first chromosomes resulting in mongolism or Down's syndrome.

Heredity also accounts for differences in temperament, in emotional tone and speed of reactions. It is also responsible for tolerance to stress reactions.

Environment is anything immediately surrounding an organism and exerts a direct influence on it. The temperature of the environment can affect the development of skin colour in certain rabbits for example.

The environmental influences are those which act upon the organism at the earlier stages of development within the mother's womb and later external environment after birth.

NEURON AND SYNAPSE

Neurons

Neurons are the basic building blocks of the nervous system. These specialized cells are the information-processing units of the brain responsible for receiving and transmitting information. Each part of the neuron plays a role in the communication of information throughout the body.

Neurons vs. Other Cells

Similarities with other cells:

- Neurons and other body cells both contain a nucleus that holds genetic information.
- Neurons and other body cells are surrounded by a membrane that protects the cell.
- The cell bodies of both cell types contain organelles that support the life of the cell, including mitochondria, Golgi bodies, and cytoplasm.

Differences that make neurons unique:

- Unlike other body cells, neurons stop reproducing shortly after birth. Because of this, some parts of the brain have more neurons at birth than later in life because neurons die but are not replaced. While neurons do not reproduce, research has shown that new connections between neurons form throughout life.
- Neurons have a membrane that is designed to sends information to other cells. The axon and dendrites are specialized structures designed to transmit and receive information. The connections between cells are known as synapses. Neurons release chemicals known as neurotransmitters into these synapses to communicate with other neurons.

The Structure of a Neuron

There are three basic parts of a neuron: the dendrites, the cell body and the axon. However, all neurons vary somewhat in size, shape, and characteristics depending on the function and role of the neuron. Some neurons have few dendritic branches, while others are highly branched in order to receive a great deal of information. Some neurons have short axons, while others can be quite long. The longest axon in the human body extends from the bottom of the spine to the big toe and averages a length of approximately three feet!

Dendrites are tree like extensions at the beginning of a neuron that help increase the surface area of the cell body and are covered with synapses. These tiny protrusions receive information from other neurons and transmit electrical stimulation to the soma.

Dendrite characteristics

- Most neurons have many dendrites.
- Short and highly branched.
- Transmits information to the cell body.

The soma is where the signals from the dendrites are joined and passed on. The soma and the nucleus do not play an active role in the transmission of the neural signal. Instead, these two structures serve to maintain the cell and keep the neuron functional.

The support structures of the cell include mitochondria, which provide energy for the cell, and the Golgi apparatus, which packages the products created by the cell and secretes them outside the cell wall.

The axon hillock is located at the end of the soma and controls the firing of the neuron. If the total strength of the signal exceeds the threshold limit of the axon hillock, the structure will fire a signal (known as an action potential) down the axon.

The axon is the elongated fiber that extends from the cell body to the terminal endings and transmits the neural signal. The larger the axon, the faster it transmits information. Some axons are covered with a fatty substance called myelin that acts as an insulator. These myelinated axons transmit information much faster than other neurons.

Axon characteristics

- Most neurons have only one axon.
- Transmit information away from the cell body.
- May or may not have a myelin covering.

The terminal buttons are located at the end of the neuron and are responsible for sending the signal on to other neurons. At the end of the terminal button is a gap known as a *synapse*. Neurotransmitters are used to carry the signal across the synapse to other neurons.

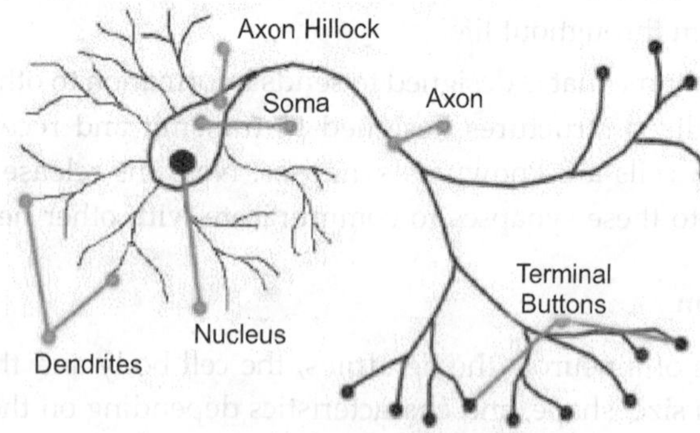

Picture showing structure of neuron

NEUROTRANSMITTER

A neurotransmitter is a chemical messenger that carries, boosts and modulates signals between neurons and other cells in the body. In most cases, a neurotransmitter is released from the axon terminal after an action potential has reached the synapse. The neurotransmitter then crosses the synaptic gap to reach the receptor site of the other cell or neuron. Then, in a process known as reuptake, the neurotransmitter attaches to the receptor site and is reabsorbed by the neuron.

Scientists do not yet know exactly how many neurotransmitters exist, but more than 100 chemical messengers have been identified. When neurotransmitters are affected by disease or drugs, there can be a number of different adverse effects on the body. Diseases such as Alzheimer's and Parkinson's are associated with deficits in certain neurotransmitters.

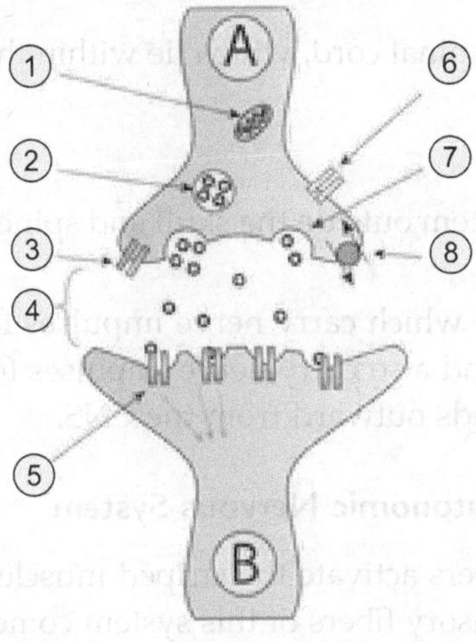

Picture showing synaptic interactions between two neurons

Types of Neurotransmitters

Neurotransmitters can be classified by function:

- **Excitatory neurotransmitters:** These types of neurotransmitters have excitatory effects on the neuron; they increase the likelihood that the neuron will fire an action potential. Some of the major excitatory neurotransmitters include epinephrine and norepinephrine.
- **Inhibitory neurotransmitters:** These types of neurotransmitters have inhibitory effects on the neuron; they decrease the likelihood that the neuron will fire an action potential. Some of the major inhibitory neurotransmitters include serotonin and GABA

Some neurotransmitters, such as acetylcholine and dopamine, can have both excitatory and inhibitory effects depending upon the type of receptors that are present.

NERVOUS SYSTEM

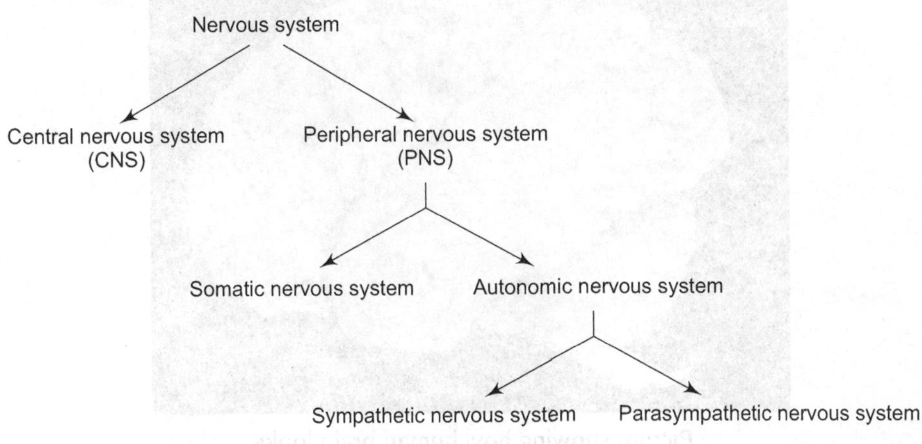

Central Nervous System and Peripheral Nervous System

CNS

It consists of the brain and the spinal cord, which lie within the bony cases of the skull and the spine.

PNS

1. The parts of the nervous system outside the skull and spine make up the peripheral nervous system.
2. PNS consists of nerve fibers which carry nerve impulses from the sensory receptors of the body inward to the CNS. And also carry nerve impulses for the movement of muscles and the excitation of certain glands outward from the CNS.

Somatic Nervous System and Autonomic Nervous System

Somatic nervous system motor fibers activate the striped muscles of the body, such as those that move arms and legs, while the sensory fibers of this system come from the major receptor organs of the body— the eyes, the ears, the touch receptors, etc.

Autonomic nervous system motor fibers activate the smooth muscles of such bodily organs as the stomach, cause secretion from certain glands such as the salivary glands and regulate the activity in the special type of muscle found in the heart. It is thus a smooth muscle, glandular and heart-muscle system.

Sympathetic Nervous System and Parasympathetic Nervous System

Sympathetic system

It is active in states of arousal and stressful situations.

Parasympathetic system

It is active in resting, quiet states.

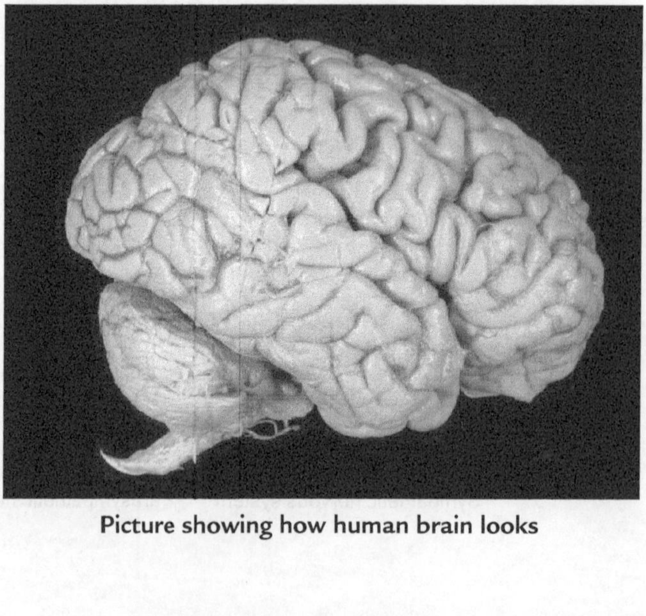

Picture showing how human brain looks

BRAIN

The brain is an extremely complex organ that can be said to give us appreciation of sensory input; serves as the originator and coordinator of motor activity; and acts as the repository for experience, intelligence, moral and social behaviour. The brain can be divided into four lobes by various sulci and gyri. The sulci (or fissures) are the grooves and the gyri are the bumps that can be seen on the surface of the brain.

The spinal cord and brain stem compose central nervous system. Brain stem consists of three subdivisions: Medulla, Pons and Midbrain. These control and regulate many bodily functions such breathing etc. They also begin the processing of sensory information from the environment and provide pathways by which this information can be carried to the forebrain. Further, no movement of the body can occur without activation of certain neurons. These are called *motoneurons.*

The **forebrain** sends nerve impulses down pathways in the spinal cord and brain stem to excite the motoneurons. Motoneurons may also be excited directly by some sensory inputs to produce simple adaptive bodily movements known as reflexes. For example rapid withdrawal of hand from fire is a reflex. Reflexes are also important in such vital activities as standing, walking and running.

Off to the back of the brain is a large, complex structure called the **cerebellum (little brain).** This structure receives sensory and other inputs from the spinal cord, brain stem and forebrain. It processes this information and then sends outputs to many parts of the brain to help make our movements precise, coordinated and smooth.

In the center or the core of the brain stem, running from the medulla up to the mid brain is a complex region containing many small clumps of neurons and a number of long and short nerve fibers. The appearance of this region reminded of early descriptive anatomists of a network. The latin word for network is a **reticulum**. Thus this region is called reticular formation. The fibers and nerve cells of the reticular formation concerned with cortical arousal are therefore known as the ascending reticular activating system (ARAS). ARAS is critically involved in regulating the various degrees of arousal—from deep sleep to alert awareness of the environment.

Most of man's awareness and conscious behaviour involves cerebral cortex. Man has a proportionately larger cortex than any other animals. The function of the cortex is broken down into motor functions, sensory functions and associative functions. Figure shows how the cerebral cortex is divided into four lobes—frontal, parietal, temporal and occipital (rear). For each lobe shown in this side view, there is a duplicate lobe in the other hemisphere of the brain.

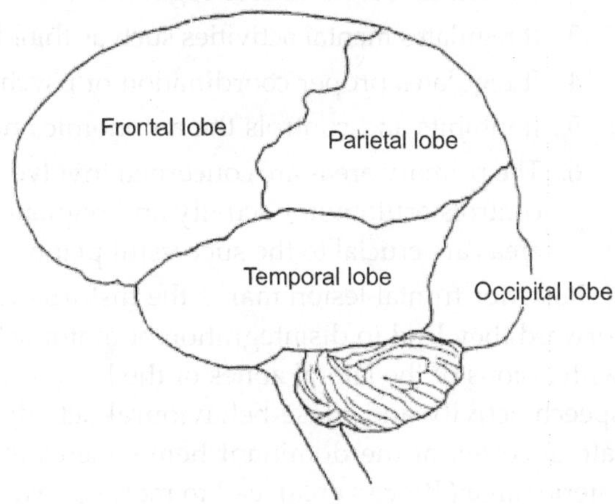

Picture showing lobes

Association Cortex

The regions in the frontal, parietal, temporal and occipital lobes are called association areas because the associations or connections between the sensory input and motor output were made in these areas. These association areas process and integrate sensory information relayed to them from the primary sensory areas of the cortex and from the thalamus; after the information has been processed, it may be sent to motor areas to be acted upon. For example, the visual association cortex of the occipital and temporal lobes receives input from the primary visual sensory cortex and processes this information, in ways as it makes it possible for us to recognize objects in the visual world.

Frontal lobe association cortex

It is the most recently developed part of the brain. In man, they make up the one third of the mass of the cerebral hemispheres. Only few decades earlier, we came to an understanding of its basic functions in many forms of human behaviour especially with regard to the regulation of complex activities. The frontal lobes lie anterior to the central sulcus and subdivided into four regions: motor area, premotor area, prefrontal area and the baso medial portion of the lobes. The frontal regions have well developed system of efferent nerve cells leading from the cortex to lower brain centres and peripheral parts of the nervous system. Luria pointed out that prefrontal regions serve as tertiary zones for the limbic system as well as for the motor system. They have rich connections with the brain stem and thalamus and all other cortical regions. Through the first set of connection prefrontal cortex particularly the basal and medial aspects of the lobes are intimately concerned with state of alertness of the organism, while the rich connections with the posterior receptor area and motor cortex allows the lateral prefrontal region to organize and execute the most complex of man's goal directed or purposive activities. From a clinical point of view, the division of prefrontal cortex into lateral and basomedial (orbitomedial) regions may serve as a useful first approximations in the search for brain behaviour relationship.

Functions of frontal lobe

1. It is responsible for planning, performance and evaluation of all motor behaviour.
2. The left frontal lobe is concerned with the functioning of the right side of the body and the right frontal lobe is concerned with the functioning of the left side of the body. This is also termed as contra-lateral regulation.
3. It regulates mental activities such as thinking, attention, memory, learning and reasoning, etc.
4. It regulates proper coordination of psychomotor activities like driving a car.
5. It inhibits and controls the autonomic and emotional response.
6. The primary areas are concerned involved in basic motor functioning; the secondary regions controls oculomotor activity and regulate general motor organization and lastly the tertiary areas are crucial to the successful planning, regulation and verification of the motor activity.

Posterior frontal lesion marks the disturbance in organization of movements. As lesions move forward they lead to disintegration of motor activities. These disturbances are marked in patients with lesions of the lateral zones of the left (dominant) frontal lobe. This is closely connected with speech activity and those behavioural acts dependent upon speech. Lesions to lower parts of lateral cortex of the dominant hemispheres lead to speech disorders. And lesions of posterior inferior area (Broca's area) lead to motor or expressive aphasia. To define the limits of Broca's area is not possible. Also lesions to anterior to broca's area will lead to speech disorder.

Prefrontal damage as a result of gunshot wounds, skull fracture etc causes changes in personality of the individual. Lack of restraint, impulsiveness, immaturity in social relationships and sometimes promiscuity in sexual behaviour characterize one personality pattern that emerges after prefrontal damage. Apathy, indifference to others, loss of initiative, decrease in spontaneous talking, and reduced emotional expression are the main features of the other patterns. The families of these patients often report that the two characteristics alternate, the patient being the euphoric for a while and then quite grouchy and touchy.

Prefrontal patients are deficient in planning courses of action; their behaviour seems to lack direction. They continue to behave in a certain way when changes in the situation demand new responses. There is a subtle memory impairment. They have trouble remembering whether one recent event occurred before or after another one.

They have difficulty with the voluntary control of their eye gaze. Without good control of voluntary gaze, prefrontal patients find certain task difficult. Their gaze is random.

Parietal lobe association cortex

Parietal lobe is the region of the cerebrum behind the central sulcus, above the lateral fissure, and in front of the occipital lobe. Parietal lobe association cortex lies behind the primary somatosensory cortex and receives inputs from visual cortex, auditory cortex, somatosensory cortex and the thalamus.

The three parts of the parietal lobe are the: postcentral gyrus, superior parietal lobule and inferior parietal lobule. Functions of parietal lobe:

1. The postcentral gyrus also known as the somatosensory cortex, receives sensory input from the contralateral half of the body. This is the primary reception area for the numerous forms of somatic sensation. Somatic sensation is made up of a number of separate modalities—among these are touch, pain, temperature, body position sense, kinetheses and vibration. Sensory impulses within the somatosensory cortex can be seen as a representation of the human body called the homunculus or the 'little man'. Neurons in this location can identify the area of the body being stimulated by the information they receive from the somatic receptors in the skin. Lesions in the postcentral gyrus result in impaired sensation from cutaneous (surface) and deep parts of the contralateral half of the body.
2. The superior parietal lobule, located caudal to the post central gyrus, lies superior to the interparietal sulcus. This lobule is regarded as an association cortex, part of which may be concerned with motor function.
3. The inferior parietal lobule (composed of the angular and supramarginal gyri) is a cortical region concerned with the integration of multiple sensory signals. Lesions in this lobule produce various syndromes of a devastating nature.
4. In the dominant hemisphere the inferior parietal area transacts mathematic functions and is closely linked to language recognition and word memory. The non-dominant parietal lobe integrates the left side of the body with its environment.
5. The postrolandic (posterior) area of the parietal lobes, integrates somesthetic stimuli for recognition and recall of form, texture and weight. Awareness of position of body parts is also generated in this area. More posterolateral areas provide accurate visual spatial relationships as well as integrate the relative perceptions with other sensations to create awareness of moving objects.

The damage to the right parietal association cortex is termed contralateral neglect. For example, the patients when asked to draw objects, they will draw only the right side ignoring the left side., they report only the touch to the right hand and some will dress only the right side of their bodies.

Problems in writing, reading and doing simple arithmetic problems often show up after the damage to the left parietal association cortex. The ability to distinguish right from left may also be impaired. Difficulty with short term verbal memory can also be a symptom of damage to left parietal association cortex. Agnosia, is a deficit in recognition ability, regardless of the sense involved. Unilateral spatial neglect is the tendency to neglect one half of the extrapersonal space in tasks like reading which require a symmetrical exploration of space. Constructional apraxia, is the difficulty in making things is also a symptom to right side damage. There are disorders of spatial cognition. Anosagnosia, is a denial of deficits or failure to perceive illness. The damage to the left side of parietal cortex includes Gerstmann's syndrome which is right left confusion, finger agnosia, agraphia and acalculia. Acalculia is a difficulty in calculating and carrying out operations of arithmetic nature (including figures and numbers. Bilateral damage causes Balint's syndrome, a visual attention and motor syndrome characterized by the inability to voluntary control of the gaze (Ocular Apraxia) and inability to integrate components of visual scene. Damage to the left parietal temporal lesions affects verbal memory and the ability to recall string of digits. Right parietal temporal lesions can produce significant changes in personality.

Temporal lobe association cortex

The temporal lobe of each hemisphere lies below the lateral fissure. Located below the lateral fissure, the temporal lobes ride between the frontal and occipital lobes, approximately at the midline of the skull, and include modules of the limbic system. They are richly connected to other lobes, the sensory system, the limbic system and the basal ganglia. The temporal lobes on either side of the brain behind the eyes and underneath the temples, store memories and images; they store our experiences.

Functions of temporal lobe

1. Amygdala is concerned with emotional control. Emotional stability is heavily influenced by this part of the brain. Optimum activity in temporal lobes enhances mood stability, while increased or decreased activity in this brain leads to fluctuating, inconsistent or unpredictable moods and behaviours.
2. Helps in understanding social cues.
3. It helps in some visual perceptions- visual object recognition and categorization.
4. It helps in language comprehension.
5. Hippocampus is the responsible for memory acquisition. It helps in retrieval of words. Essential components of memory are integrated and stored in temporal lobes.

Auditory agnosia is the difficulty in recognizing melodies or problems in distinguishing non-language sounds from one another may result from damage to the temporal lobe association areas. Since portions of temporal association cortex receive inputs from the visual areas of the brain in the occipital lobe, various visual agnosias can follow temporal lobe damage.

Another Disorder is Impaired Attention

The left temporal lobe contains a region of association cortex called Wernicke's area. Damage to this region markedly impairs the understanding of speech and written language. Speech is however fluent but conveys little meaning.

Occipital lobes

It forms the most posterior portions of the cerebral hemisphere, at the back of the head. Therefore, they are not vulnerable to injury because of their location. It occupies only a small portion of the total brain, so its functions are somewhat limited than other areas. Occipital lobes are the centre of our visual perception system.

Functions of occipital lobes

1. They are involved in understanding of visual images and written words.
2. They are responsible for transferring visual information to other parts of the brain.
3. Projections from occipital lobes to the superior temporo-parietal area are important for perceiving motion of objects.
4. Areas in the inferior temporal visual association cortex are important for recognition of colour and shape as well as the recognition of faces.

Damage to this area of brain lead to many defects, such as: cerebral blindness, hysterical blindness, dyslexia, colour blindness and problems in perceiving faces or objects. Alexia without agraphia also occurs. It is also known as pure alexia, word form alexia. It is a reading difficulty that consists of a failure to recognize words without evidence of dysphasia. Visual hallucinations are described frequently in conditions affecting temporo-occipital or parieto – occipital regions.

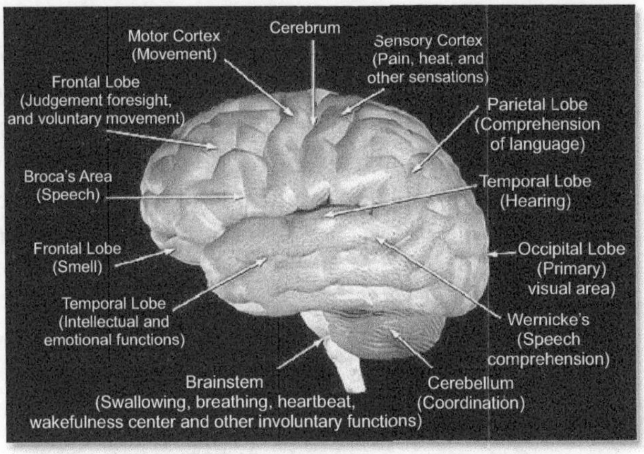

Picture showing the brain lobes and other various parts

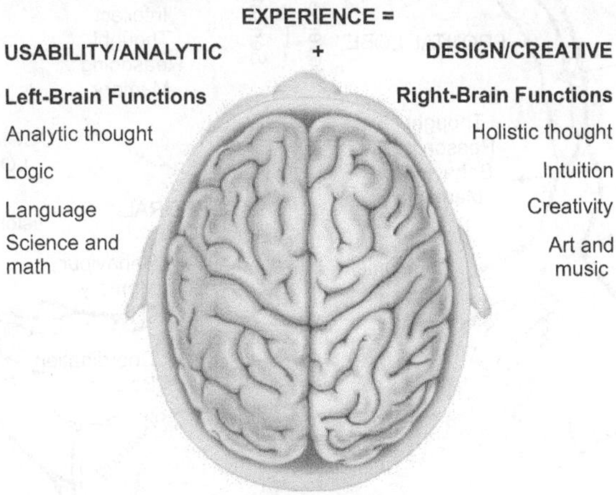

Picture showing left and right hemispheres

Left Hemisphere and Right Hemisphere

Left hemisphere

1. Left hemisphere is the centre for understanding language, formulating language for communication and thinking with language symbols.

2. The left brain is said to be the analytical, logical, mathematical hemisphere, concerned with cause and effect scientific thinking.

Right hemisphere

1. Right hemisphere is usually specialized to deal with images, spatial relationships and pattern recognition. However left hemisphere has some spatial abilities and the right hemisphere has some language capabilities.
2. The right brain is essential for the kind of thinking that goes into the creation of painting or musical composition.
3. People with left hemisphere strokes (right-sided paralysis) are much more likely to have serious language problems than are people with right hemisphere strokes (left-sided paralysis).
4. Left hemisphere has wernicke's area, involved in understanding of spoken and written language. It also plays an important role in formulation of sentences— figuring out what we want to say or write and selecting words to express it. The left hemisphere also has a broca area. Damage to this area, induces a slow speech with great effort; articulation of sounds of speech poorly; tending to omit pronouns, adjectives, adverbs and articles; uses the singular of nouns; and has great trouble with the tense of verbs. The angular gyrus is important in the brain processes involved in reading. Damage to this region leads to dyslexia, *i.e.*, Patients may be able to communicate and understand speech but they cannot read.

A Comprehensive Picture of Human Brain

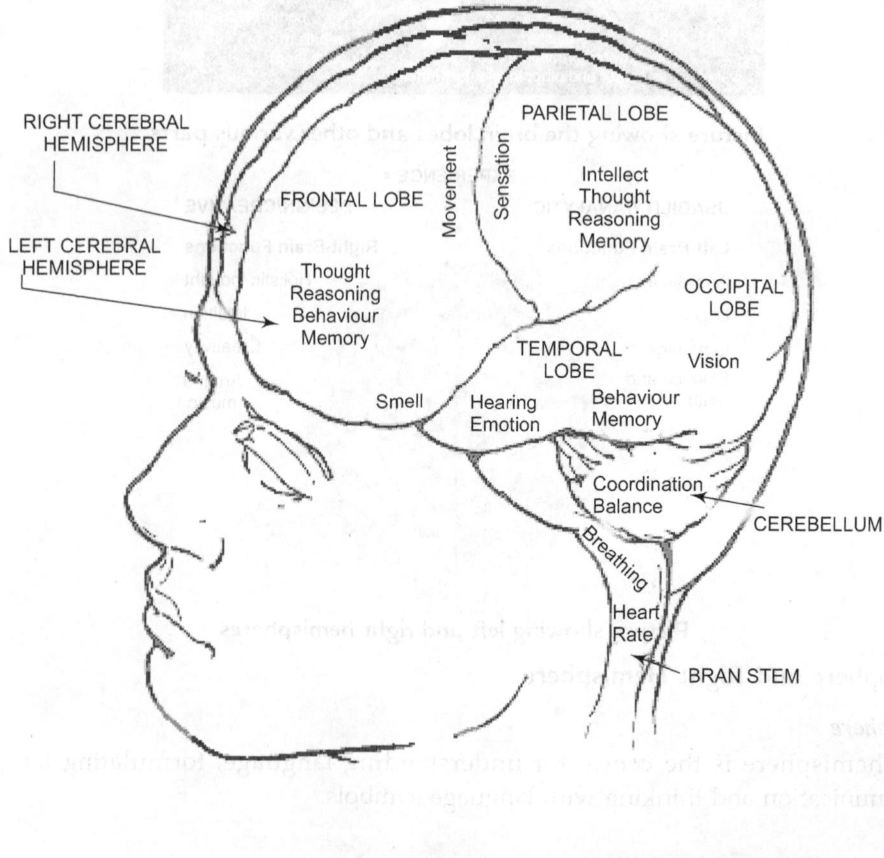

GLANDULAR CONTROLS OF BEHAVIOUR

The body is integrated by organization of cells into tissues, organs and systems activities by the nervous system and endocrine glands whose chemical secretions may have similar effects in widely separated locations in the body. Glands are organs made up of various tissues that help in secretions of substances that carried and needed throughout the body. A gland is a group of cells that produces and secretes, or gives off, chemicals. A gland selects and removes materials from the blood, processes them and secretes the finished chemical product for use somewhere in the body. Some types of glands release their secretions in specific areas.

There are two types of glands exocrine glands which are duct glands as they secrete into a duct or pipeline that carries the secretions to their destination. It can be the digestive tract, surface of the body. The second type of gland is endocrine or ductless. Their secretions are directly into the bloodstream. The secretions of endocrine glands are called hormones.

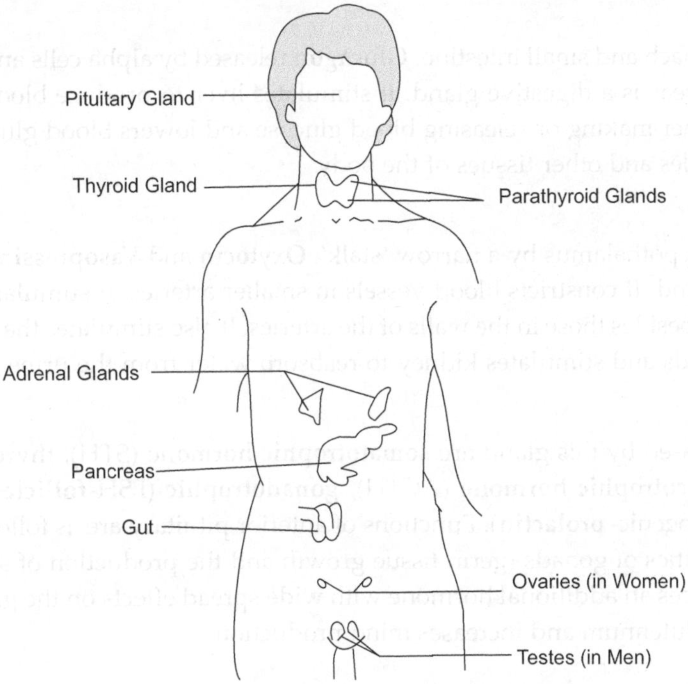

Endocrine System

DESCRIPTIONS OF VARIOUS GLANDS AND FUNCTIONS

Thyroid gland

It lies on both sides of the wind pipe, below the voice box. Hormone released by this gland is **thyroxin**. It is necessary for maintaining energy and activity. It raises the metabolism of the body.

Parathyroid gland

It is a pea shaped gland attached to the thyroid gland. Hormone released by this gland is **parathormone**. It is necessary to control the calcium level and calcium to phosphate ratio required for normal nerve and muscle cell functioning.

Adrenal cortex

They are located on top of the kidney. **Corticoids** are the hormones released by adrenal cortex gland. They regulate the sodium and potassium balance of the body. They promoted sodium retention and potassium loss through the kidneys. Further, they increase carbohydrate metabolism to raise basal metabolic rate. It produces both male sex hormone – androgen and female sex hormone – estrogen. It plays a pivotal role in sexual functioning.

Adrenal medulla

It is located in the autonomic nervous system. **Norepinephrine** and **epinephrine** are the hormones released by adrenal medulla gland. Norepinephrine raises the blood pressure by constricting the arteries. Epinephrine raises the blood pressure by accelerating the heart rate. Epinephrine stimulates anterior pituitary gland to secrete ACTH, which in turn stimulates the release of corticoids from the adrenal cortex.

Pancreas

It lies between stomach and small intestine. **Glucagon** released by alpha cells and **insulin** released by beta cells. Pancreas is a digestive gland. It stimulates liver to produce blood glucose. Insulin inhibits liver in either making or releasing blood glucose and lowers blood glucose by increasing its use by the muscles and other tissues of the body.

Posterior pituitary

It is connected to hypothalamus by a narrow 'stalk'. **Oxytocin** and **Vasopressin** are the hormones released by this gland. It constricts blood vessels in smaller arteries. It stimulates the contraction of smooth muscles besides those in the walls of the arteries. It also stimulates the ejection of milk by the mammary glands and stimulates kidney to reabsorb water from the urine.

Anterior pituitary

The hormones released by this gland are **somatotrophic hormone** (STH), **thyrotrophic hormone** (TTH), **adrenocorticotrophic hormone** (ACTH), **gonadotrophic** (FSH-**follicle stimulating**, LH-**luteinzing** and lactogenic–**prolactin**). Functions of anterior pituitary are as follows. It controls the thyroid, three activities of gonads (germ tissue growth and the production of sex and pregnancy hormone). It produces an additional hormone with wide spread effects on the growth of the body. It develops corpus lutennum and increases mind production.

Gonads

Androgens and **Estrogen** are the two hormones released by this gland. It is responsible for fertility and secondary sex characteristics of the body.

Pineal gland

It lies on the top of the posterior part of the third ventricle of the brain. **Melatonin** is released by this gland. It acts to bleach the skin pigment cells and suppresses the activity of gonads. It regulates the timing of menstrual cycle in man as well as in animals.

Thymus gland

It lies between the breastbone and the heart. **Lymphocytes** are the secretions of this gland. It helps in combating disease bacteria and react to the presence of foreign proteins. It produces antibodies that neutralize disease bacteria and viruses.

MUSCULAR CONTROL OF BEHAVIOUR

The physiological activities and behaviours are performed by muscles. Muscles are involved in internal and external movement of the body. Like walking, running, smiling and showing aggression, excretion and circulation. These kinds of behaviour are exhibited by contracting and relaxing of the muscle. Smooth muscles respond to appropriate stimuli in a reflexive or involuntary manner. The coordination and control of muscles determine the precision, speed and strength of motor performance. After exercise and prolonged stimulation, muscles lose contractibility and regain their rigour through rest.

REFLECT YOURSELF

1. Elucidate upon the structure of neuron.
2. Discuss muscular and glandular controls of behaviour.
3. Discuss the functioning of all the lobes of the human brain.

3

ATTENTION

TOPICS COVERED IN THIS CHAPTER
• Process of Attention • Characteristics of Attention • Factors Affecting Attention

PROCESS OF ATTENTION

In our day to day lives we get exposed to many potential stimuli but we perceive relatively a few of them at any given time. We do not react equally to all the stimuli in our environment, instead we focus on few. The concentration of awareness on certain objects and events or stimuli ignoring others in the environment is referred to as attention.

For example, if one is looking for MBA course from a private university, he/she will get hold of eye of the billboard, honking, traffic and other potential stimuli in the environment.

According to **Zimbardo**, attention is defined as "A state of focussed awareness accompanied by central nervous system readiness to respond to stimulation." The process of attention also involves: (a) adjustment of sense organs (b) adjustment of posture (c) muscle tension. If one is asked to examine the picture which he/she has not seen as yet, you will notice the movement of eyes, the change in his posture, tightening of muscles on the face as he tries to identify the picture. Other physiological changes however are not observable such as changes in heart beat, electrical activity of the skin.

CHARACTERISTICS OF ATTENTION

- Attention is never fixed, liable to shift and fluctuate noted by **Woodworth** and **Schlosberg** (1954). Shifting is generally accounted for by fatigue, adaptation, and satiation. This is *SHIFT* OF ATTENTION.

- Attention can be active or passive. Active attention is voluntary (students attending to a lecture). Passive attention is involuntary. This is DISTRACTION OF ATTENTION. (dropping of a book)
- Attention is physiologically related.
- The process of attention divide our field of experience into a focus and a margin. This focus shifts from time to time. This is SELECTIVE ATTENTION.
- Attention is selective but shortlived. SPAN OF ATTENTION refers to the numbers of objects, letters and digits one can attend in a fraction of a second so short as to exclude eye movement or counting. It is the amount of information an observer can grasp from a complex stimulus at a single, momentary exposure. For example, the eyewitness who saw the speeding truck, running over the victim, reports the number to the police.
- When an individual detects and respond to a target or signal which usually occurs infrequently over a period of time. This is VIGILANCE OF ATTENTION. Example, soldiers posted at the border locates a foreign plane in their territory.
- Attention can be allocated differently to different tasks. This is DIVISION OF ATTENTION. The concept of division of attention involve simultaneous focussing of attention on two separate objects. However, simultaneous performance on two attentive tasks involve cognition does not ordinarily occur. For example, you ask your friend to draw circles while saying counting from 0 to 100.

FACTORS AFFECTING ATTENTION

Factors which determine which stimuli will gain our attention. These factors can be classified into:

External Factors

1. **Nature:** By nature of stimulus is meant whether the stimulus is visual or auditory. Normally a picture with human beings or inanimate objects attracts attention more readily than words.
2. **Novelty:** Any unusual or irregular event is liable to gain more attention. Objects, sounds, smells and tastes to which one is accustomed may go unnoticed but one will observe a strange stimulus immediately.
3. **Intensity:** A brilliantly lighted sign or the tone of a loudspeaker attract attention more rapidly than a dim lighted sign or a low tone from a record player.
4. **Location:** The best location of a visual stimulus for attracting attention is directly in front of the eyes in the centre of the page. Objects on the periphery of visual sensation some-times fail to get noticed.
5. **Contrast:** Things which are different from their surroundings or those that contrast with others in the surroundings are more readily attended to the others.
6. **Size:** The physical dimension or size of the stimulus also influences attention. Normally if two stimuli are competing for an individual's attention, he/she will notice the one that is bigger. A word with the low case letters among a group of capital letters may get greater attention than the word in capital letters. For example : Lion. Here too contrast is involved.

7. **Colour:** Some colours get more attention than others. Here, contrast plays an important role. An individual is interested in more of a coloured backgrounds than in grey and he/she normally pays more attention to red and white designs in preference to black and white.
8. **Movement:** A moving object usually gets more attention than a stationary one.
9. **Repetition:** When a particular stimulus is repeated several times one may ultimately notice it, though it failed to gain attention initially.

Internal Factors

- Mental set of the subject refers to the situation where the tuning of one's mind may put the individual to look at the problem in a particular way repeatedly and hence failing in solving the problem.
- Bodily state of the subject: A sick person may not notice a bright stimulus as compared to a fit person.
- Meaningful of the material: Meaningful material is likely to be well noticed than the nonsense.

REFLECT YOURSELF

1. Discuss the nature of attention.
2. Discuss the factors affecting attention.

4

PERCEPTION

TOPICS COVERED IN THIS CHAPTER

- Introduction
- Process of Perception
- Characteristics of Perception

INTRODUCTION

Whenever the sense organs receive certain stimuli they are generally processed to make them meaningful. A stimulus has different meanings for different people. The same event may be perceived differently by different people who attend to it. It may be meaningful to all but may have somewhat different meaning for each individual. A single individual can also perceive the same stimulus, pattern differently on different occasions. According to **Hilgard** and **Atkinson**, perception is the process of becoming aware of objects, qualities or relations by the way of the sense organs.

PROCESS OF PERCEPTION

Various physical energies act in the environment. They in turn act on sensory receptors of an individual. When these receptors get activated the nerve impulses travel to the brain. During this transformation of various information, the physical responses of the sense organs are first translated into a compatible form with the nerve impulses which are previously received and stored so that the incoming impulse are tallied with the past experience.

The minimal level of physical energy necessary to excite and to produce response in a given individual is called absolute threshold. The process of converting physical energy of the stimulus into impulses so that the nervous system can transmit to the brain is called transduction. **Sensory processes:** channels through which a person comes to know about the world around him/her are his/her senses. Sensation occurs when any of the sense organs receive a stimulus from the external or internal environment of the individual. Each of the sense organ is stimulated by a specific and different form of external and internal energy.

CHARACTERISTICS OF PERCEPTION

- **Different meaning:** Stimulus has different meaning for different people. This is because of perception of same stimuli varies from person to person. Perceptual view is different from person to person as past experiences also differ because all individuals may not be exposed to same kind of environment.
- **Interpretation** of meaning depends on many factors. It is necessary to interpret selected sensations in light of the past experiences of the individual in order to determine the meaning of the perceptual experience.
- **Interpretation of stimulus** is influenced by various factors. Such as—different objects in their appropriate identity and form—past experience—stimulating circumstances—present psychological need of a person.
- **Factors affecting perception past experiences with stimuli:** An individual past experience and learning affect his/her present perception. It is because that an object acquires different meanings for different persons depending upon one's past experience.
- **Learning:** Learning itself is based on past experience. Aspects of perception depend upon learning. For example, size constancy develops as a result of learning, varies from child to an adult.
- **Motivation and emotion:** This factor plays an important role in affecting perception as stimuli are perceived in terms of one's drives (motivation), interest, values and needs (emotion). Sensory deprivation results in the individual's ability to make adaptive perceptual discrimination. Such deprivation cause hallucination. Hallucination is a perception of stimulus that is absent in the given environment.
- **Maturation:** Helps in relearning all the auditory and tactile association to accommodate the new visual frame of reference.

REFLECT YOURSELF

1. Discuss the factors affecting perception.
2. What is the process of perception?

5

LEARNING

TOPICS COVERED IN THIS CHAPTER

- Introduction
- Learning Curve
- Theories of Learning
- Factors Affecting Learning
- Transfer of Learning
- Determine Your Learning Style
- How to Make Learning Happen?

INTRODUCTION

Sarah learned typing when she was in school. When she got married her husband got cancer. Because of changed circumstances, her attitude towards expenses and life in general changed. Here, in this example we notice change in behaviour towards life as well learning of typing skill is also noticeable. What is learning? What is the importance of this cognitive process? Learning refers to a relatively permanent change in behaviour which occurs as a result of prior experience. Other definitions are : "learning refers to changes in behaviour potential as well as to changes in overt behaviour," for example: by studying a map we might learn the route to a friends home without actually going there. Since the potential for such behaviour would now exist, whereas, it did not exist before, learning is said to have occurred. The third definition say learning is reserved for changes in behaviour stemming from experience—our interactions with the world around us. Changes derived from factors such as fatigue, physical growth or recovery from injury are not viewed as instances of learning. According to cognitive psychologists "learning refers to a change in thinking the way information is processed which occurs as a result of prior experience," according to them learning is a cognitive proces which originates from perception *i.e.,* deriving meaning to a stimulus. That is why learning is central to human behaviour. As, entire socialization depends upon learning. Moreover, it leads to—development of personality—development of skills,—include processes such as effective observation, acquisition, retention and application of knowledge and skills,—acquiring appropriate forms of emotional expressions, and control,—development of interests and ways of thinking,—development of preferences, prejudices and attitudes.

Characteristics of Learning

Learning is a continuous process: an individual spends the major part of his/her lifetime in learning. It takes place outside home, school, college, workplace through one's contacts with people objects and events. Learning is a gradual process, it takes time to learn an activity properly. Learning is a process spread over a period of time. One may find difficult to learn any activity in the beginning but through his/her continous efforts one may learn. One may reach a level of competence in motor skills but not in learning abstract concepts such as literature, history as there is no physiological limit. Learning is different from performance because performance depends upon learning. Until and unless learning takes place, performance cannot take place. Level of learning determines level of performance. Secondly, performance depends upon learning and learning depends upon stimulus conditions and motivation. Learnt behaviour is different from behaviour attributed to maturation. Because, what he/she learns depends to a great extent upon the nature of his/her environment and experience. Whether a person is interested in physics or geography, whether she likes his/her school, whether she is conservative or liberal in her social attitudes. Whether she is honest and she studies well or keeps away from studies are determined to a ' great extent by the nature of his/her experience. Reflex action and instinctive behaviour are different from learnt behaviour. Instincts are complex behavioural patterns that appear at different stages of maturation and development. Eg. Eating behaviour of persons and building of nests by birds. Reflex behaviour is direct and immediate response of a muscle or a gland to the stimulation of a sense organ. E.g. blinking of eyes in response to sudden movement in front of a person. These are innate tendencies which are not acquired through practice.

LEARNING CURVE

Learning curve consists of a number of irregularities as progress is not constant. The fluctuations are due to—in attention, fatigue, loss of interest and changes in physical conditions.

The rate of learning—is measured by performance, varies from person to person and varies from time to time. Learning curve has five stages:

1. **Period of slow progress:** generally when a person learns a new activity early progress is slow. This is due to the fact that the learner has to master such skills before he can put together a complete performance or he has to unlearn conflicting skills or habits e.g. If a person is learning typing he first learns the basic operations like position of different keys , setting the paper and adjusting movements of fingers. In some case there is a rapid rise in the progress due to positive transfer of a previous learnt activity, initial enthusiasm for learning a new activity and early phases of the total activity are the easiest.
2. **Period of rapid rise:** In this stage learner's output rises rapidly. It ordinarily learner's catching on the purpose and nature of the task. In typewriting once the learner had learnt the coordination of fingers shows rapid progress.

3. **Plateau (no visible progress):** Learning curve is frequently displaced by what is called as plateau period of no apparent progress which is followed by further gains. Thus, in typewriting making a consistent effort a person may reach a point perhaps for weeks no further progress is made such periods are proceeded and followed by improvement are called plateau.
4. **Period of sudden rise:** At the end of plateau learner acquires better techniques which help in later on to show rapid progress. The ups and downs may continue because of changes.
5. **Leveling off:** All learning may finally slow down and reach a level where there is no improvement. No one can continue to improve indefinitely in a given situation. The learning curve will reach the limit when no further improvement is passed on. This limit is known as physiological limit. It is that degree of ability which a particular individual cannot surpass because of absolute inherited limits in the speed of motor or mental response. The task has certain limitations. Different individuals have different upper limits inherent limitations. Ordinarily a person stays at a level ....which may be called as practical level reached by us in different skills are far moved from the physiological limits. Normally a person with speed and efficiency are below their maximum possibility under specific incentives such as keen competitions, bonus in pay, award for scholarship. In learning of abstract material such as law, history, literature there is no physiological ability. As there is possibility to learn more.

THEORIES OF LEARNING

Trial and Error Learning

Trial and error learning was given by E. L. Thorndike. Correct responses are learnt as a result of their reward or punishment. Incorrect responses are eliminated. Following laws were formulated. Thorndike conducted an experiment on cats. He took a cat and locked in a cage. Lever was inside the cage, it was such, that it could reach mental capacity of the organism. The cat was hungry and food was kept out side, cat started scratching, leaping, jumping and clawing the cage in order to get the food. These random activities continued for some time. During the agitating movements made by the hungry cat, the lever got pressed. She quickly reached to the food. She was again locked inside the cage. This happened for several trials. Gradually the number of errors reduced and ultimately cat learnt to get out of the cage. This happended because at the end there was an attractive reward which became cause of learning.

Characteristic features of this experiment

- Cat was hungry, restless, indulged in random activities.
- She had an exploratory behaviour. Looking for ways to achieve its goal. The way was not clear.
- Eventually in the course of activities, by chance the lever got pressed. The door opened. It was allowed to eat little bit and returned to the cage.
- On the subsequent trials cat improved and reduce the random activities. As trials continued the cat eliminated useless activities. Finally she learnt to press the lever, as soon as it was put in a cage to make further attempt.
- Gradual reduction in the errors and time.

(a) **Law of effect:** it implies the satisfaction of the motive which act as cause of further learnt behaviour. This law can be explained with the help of this experiment. Some rats were put into the maze with no incentive except their natural curiosity. There times of getting out were found of irregular but fairly long. After a few trials, the food dish was introduced at the exit and therefore the time curves began to fall sharply.

(b) **Law of intensity:** it implies that the greater the size of reward and stronger the motivation the faster and surer is learning experiment. Eight groups of mice learnt to find food in a simple maze varying delays between correct choice and the food. A tendency was seen for learning to be most efficient when a short-time elapsed between the response and reward.

(c) **Law of exercise:** the bond b/w the stimulus and response is strengthened when S-R association is established and repeated for in the formation of habits. Further two laws were formed.

(d) **Law of use:** implies that when a learnt behaviour is still in practice it maintains continuity and revision of the learnt behaviour. E.g. learn to wash hands before meal is taught to small children but this habit becomes automatic during a gradual period of time.

(e) **Law of disuse:** implies that the learnt behaviour is not in practice thus it loses its accuracy in verbal or motor skill though leaving a faint impression upon the memory. E.g. learning a nursery rhyme.

Classical Conditioning

The term classical means in the established manner and conditioning means simple modification of behaviour. Thus, classical conditioning means simple modification of behaviour in a established manner. This concept was first laid by Russian psychologist, Ivan Pavlov. He did an experiment, where a hungry dog was locked inside the cage. It was noted that with the sight of food pellet, he salivated. Now salivation is a unconditioned response and food is a unconditioned stimulus. A few trials later, bell, a neutral stimulus was paired with food pellet. It was found that now dog has started salivating even at the sound of bell. This was conditioned response. But this conditioned response weakened when bell was sounded alone without food pellet. As soon as food was introduced again, spontaneous recovery took place.

Characteristics of classical conditioning

- Classical conditioning is a form of associative learning. That is, it is one form of associative learning where a connection between a stimulus and a response is established. Eg. behaviour of a child who avoids burning firewood after being burnt by it once. *i.e.,* he/she forms an association between fire and pain (reflected through reflex action).
- Classical conditioning includes a variety of experience *i.e.,* it includes both pleasant and unpleasant experiences. e.g. pleasant experience, one like sing a song not because it is melodious but it is associated with some pleasant experience. And unpleasant experience, vomiting associated with eating of spoilt bread. The child may dislike bread throughout his life.
- Classical conditioning involves substitution and association of one stimulus for another. *i.e.,* according to Pavlov, CC is defined as automatization of behaviour by repetition of stimuli which accompany a given response and which ultimately become a cause for the behaviour

which formerly they had accompanied. I.e. Individual learns to respond to the second stimulus in the same way as one responds to the first stimulus. e.g. Dog learnt to salivate at the sound of the bell.

Significance of classical conditioning

- One special application of classical conditioning procedures is in the development of bladder control of the euretic child.
- It is also used to determine the sensory capacities of infants. To help them in speech and auditory therapy in handicapped persons.
- It is involved in formation of attitudes and emotional reactions.
- Classical conditioning accounts for much incidental learning in one's every day.
- Through classical conditioning one learn to respond to signals, alarms and warnings.
- It is readily seen in training an animal to perform an activity.

Operant Conditioning

In instrumental conditioning, an action of the learner is instrumental in bringing about a change in the environment that makes the action more or less likely to occur again in the future. It is an active process, in which the learner responds in such way in which his response affects the stimuli. It involves voluntary behaviour, in which response are controlled by the individual. This process is seen in human learning. Response reinforcing stimulus association depends on the consequence of responding. Here, the reinforcement follows the response because it is contingent upon the occurrence of the response. This concept was given by B.F. Skinner.

Characteristics of operant conditioning

- Response is instrumental in getting the reward or escaping punishment. The organism learns to make a response which means achieving a goal. The response can be instrumental in getting a reward or a positive incentive. (e.g. pressing the lever to get food) or it could be a means of avoiding or escaping from an annoying experience or a negative incentive such as moving away hand from fire.
- In instrumental conditioning the reinforcement is contingent on the response. E.g. Suppose while playing within a tin container, the child finds chocolate and starts eating it.
- Learnt response is not elicited by specifiable stimulus. In operant conditioning "to be learnt" response is not elicited by a specifiable stimulus. In instrumental conditioning the naturally occurring responses emitted by the organism are strengthened by reinforcement.

Significance of operant conditioning

- Operant conditioning is used to shape desired behaviour, initiating speech to psychotic patient.
- Once a operant response is established this conditioning helps in investigating the factors affecting organism. These are brain disturbances, physiological conditions, variations in reinforcement.
- Operant conditioning helps us to understand the amount of reinforcement involved in conditioned or unconditioned response of a person.
- The person's beliefs, customs and traditions are learnt through operant conditioning.

- Instrumental conditioning includes positive reinforcement which helps in clinical and educational research, control of alcoholism and control of deviant children.

Similarity Between Classical and Operant Conditioning

Generalization of stimulus is the tendency to give conditioned responses to stimuli that are similar in some way to the conditioned stimulus but have never been paired with unconditioned stimulus. The greater the similarity of these stimuli to the original conditioned stimulus, the greater the amount of generalization. **Stimulus discrimination** discrimination is the process of learning to make one response to one stimulus and another response—or no response. In classical conditioning, discrimination are developed in classical conditioning by pairing one stimulus with an unconditioned stimulus and never pairing another stimulus with an unconditioned stimulus. In operant conditioning, discrimination are developed when differences in reinforcement accompany different stimuli. Stimulus discrimination in instrumental conditioning is referred to as the stimulus control of behaviour. **Reinforcement** a reinforce is any stimulus that strengthens or maintains the occurrence of a behaviour. In classical conditioning, the UCS elicits the response to be learnt and also functions as the reinforce. In instrumental, a reinforce is any stimulus or stimulus situation that strengthens the response which preceeds it. At the sight of every child is conditioned to look for chocolate. **Extinction** is a process of learning to inhibit the response acquired in conditioning. In classical conditioning, extinction of a classically conditioned response is defined as a decrease in the strength of a CR as a result of repeatedly eliciting it in the absence reinforcement. If at the sound of a conditioned stimulus (bell) UCS food is not presented *(reinforcer) the conditioned response is likely to become extinct. In operant conditioning,* similar process takes place in similar way. I.e. when reinforcement is no more contingent on the response. **Spontaneous recovery** is a process of reappearance of CR spontaneously. Extinction does not completely erase conditioning. If reconditioning is done it is much faster than the original conditioning. This process is seen in classical as well as operant conditioning.

Cognitive Approach

Cognitive approach is modern approach to learning. According to cognitive psychologists "learning refers to a change in thinking , the way information is processed which occurs as a result of prior experience." According to cognitive approach learning is a cognitive process which originates from perception (i.e., deriving meaning to a stimulus). unlike behaviourists who explained only stimulus response association, cognitive psychologists explain S-0-R what mental process function after receiving stimulus and before evolving a response. These mental processes include —problem solving and reasoning, acquisition of a large information, change in perception, new information is stored and old information comes to have new meanings and associations as a result of past experience. The cognitive psychologists opposed the view of behaviourists that learning can be better understood in terms of external or environment. But Edward C.Tolman study reveals that overt behaviour is not necessary for learning to occur. There are two types of learning:

Imitation

Individuals limitate others in order to become a part of the social group. He watches, hears someone else do or say and then attempts to copy his behaviour in this way individuals acquire many of their characteristics in this manner.

Insight learning

Insight is defined as sudden perception of relationship between the learner, the goal and intervening obstacles. Insight occurs when the learner suddenly sees the relations and the relevant associations involved in a task and is able to solve the problem immediately. Kohler experiment show that how chimpanzee tries with smaller stick then with bigger stick to obtain the bananas which were hung out of his reach. The chimpanzee solved the problem which show that it had some insight. Through this experiment it get proved that solution was sudden rather than being the result of a gradual trial and error process. Secondly, once chimpanzee solved a problem these after it was able to solve the problem again with few irrelevant moves as unlike a rat which continues to make irrelevant responses in the skinner box for many trials.

Conclusion—instead chimpanzee's solution reflect a mental trial and error, *i.e.*, animals form a mental representation of the problem. Learning cannot be same for all species , as insight learning takes place in higher order species like humans and chimpanzee's because every specie has its own capacity to receive problem and solve it. Secondly, lower order species cannot readily transfer what they had learnt to a novel situation. This is proved by Kohlers experiment. Kohler chimpanzee sultan stacked some boxes strewn around him, climbed the "platform" and grabbed the bananas, which were too high for him. Cognitive approach found that animals and human beings can acquire new responses and information through exposure to the actions of others. Thish is observational learning. Observational learning is more complex than imitation because imitation is blind copying of behaviour, which is found in smaller children and chimpanzee. In a zoo, one may find chimpanzee smoking a cigarette. Smaller children saying dialogues of movies without knowing the actual meaning of it. Observational learning was studied by B andura. He found that 1st stage is attention, extract certain features of model, encode it and store it and then convert this memory representation into action. Further, it takes place when if the model is seen to have some reinforcing consequence, if model has high social status, something common between imitator and model, attend to model's behaviour and store in LTM and later bring it to use and imitation also depends on imitator's own capacity.

FACTORS AFFECTING LEARNING

Feedback: or knowledge of results if provided at every step helps in learning and maintaining interest through competence. **Distribution of practice:** even distribution of practice and rest periods benefit a lot in verbal and motor learning. **Whole and part learning:** whole learning is more efficient than part learning as it does not interrupt the continuity of the learning and meaning of the matter is not lost but depending upon the length of the content which is to be learnt. **Meaningfulness:** meaningful and relevant matter makes the learning move rapid as fewer number of trials or practice is given to this process. **Interest and aptitude:** if an individual has interest on a particular subject he/she learn faster and if he/she knows that it is worthwhile and will lead to the attainment of his/her goal. **Motivation:** refers to the state within a person that drives behaviour towards some goal. Both directing and energizing features play an important role in learning.

TRANSFER OF LEARNING

Learning is a serial and interactional process. The effect of past learning on a new learning is taken as transfer. It also means carrying over. Learning of one skill when extended and utilized in another field is one aspect of transfer. By transfer of training is meant spread of learning. The transfer takes place in motor, intellectual, emotional spheres. Transfer of training is readily observable in motor skills.

Theories of Transfer of Learning

Theory of formal discipline

It is an old theory based on faculty psychology. According to this theory a faculty or power is developed by exercise just as a muscle is developed. Subjects to be taught in school should be selected not based on their practical application. Subjects like latin, geometry were taught for the purpose of strengthening the reasoning faculty and power of observation, comparison and synthesis.

Theory of identical components or elements

According to this theory transfer is possible only when there is similarity or resemblance between the two situations. Situations in which learning took place and to which it is to be transferred. Thorndike and Woodworth have carried out experimental investigation. Thorndike is of the opinion that transfer depends upon how much identical elements of content, attitude or methods were found common in both situations.

Theory of transfer of principles or generalization

This theory considers the criteria of insight as basis of transfer. Charles N. Judd concluded that learning with full grasp with scientific generalization or learning in which the learner has gained a view of a wide- range of relations is capable of being transferred to situations that are different from those in which he was first trained. The theory maintains that transfer is possible not because of objective identities b/w the two learning tasks but because of the appropriate application of the principles and generalisation learnt in the old situations.

Transfer as stimulus—response analysis

It is advocated by experimentalists. Poffer Berger based it on his experiments and the results are: (A) when there are no identical bonds between the stimulus and response in the two processes, the influence of one test upon another will be neither positive nor negative neither beneficial nor detrimental. (B) when a given process involves one or more bonds, previously formed, there will be positive transfer effect. (C) when one process necessitates the breaking of previously formed bonds and forming new ones there will be negative effect.

DETERMINE YOUR LEARNING STYLE

A. **An active learner:** Likes to apply the lesson in real life. Likes to discuss the lessons with others what they have learned. Enjoys discussions and group problem solving.

B. A **reflective learner:** Needs time to process the lessons learned. Needs to see the forest as well as the trees. Appreciates it when there is a pause after learning.

C. A **factual learner:** Loves to learn facts and easily remember names and faces Prefers concrete details.

D. A **theoretical learner:** Is good at seeing the forest. Does not like repetition and fact based learning is comfortable with abstractions.

E. A **visual learner** Recalls details in terms of pictures and images. Prefers the use of pictures in lessons in reading books, she/he pays more attention to pictures than words.

F. A **verbal learner:** Recalls details in terms of words in reading texts, she/he focuses more on the words.

G. A **linear learner:** Likes to solve problems step by step learns better if the details are presented on the list. Learns best when the material is sequenced from the easiest to the hardest.

H. A **holistic learner:** Likes to piece together the lessons

Learns better if the materials are presented as a whole story with details.

In solving math problems, she/he sees the solution but agonizes over the steps for the solution.

HOW TO MAKE LEARNING HAPPEN?

1. Avoid procrastination
2. Avoid bad influence
3. Avoid distractions
4. Avoid becoming pessimistic
5. Avoid laziness

REFLECT YOURSELF

1. Discuss theories of learning.
2. Discuss the stages in learning curve.
3. Elucidate upon different learning styles.
4. Write a short note on transfer of learning.
5. What are the differences between classical conditioning and instrumental conditioning?

6

MEMORY

TOPICS COVERED IN THIS CHAPTER

- Introduction
- Different Conceptualizations of Human Memory
- Forgetting
- Current State of Research on Memory
- Mnemonics

INTRODUCTION

Memory is the ability to recall or remember information, events or skills learnt in the past. The term information refers to some news on TV or any information on billboards. Events could be death of a loved one or any happy moment like attending a Christmas carnival. Skills could be the soft skills or learning of hard skills.

The sequence followed in the process of memory is registration, retention, recall and recognition. Memory is a mental processes involving in storing and retrieving information. They originate in perception or experiences. Experiences have some kind of trace behind (in perception). Memories differ in content and context from person to person of any same situation. Memory is by no means a complete record of all events in our life. Memories are rarely exact copies of earlier experiences. What we store and retrieve is influenced by factors (physical health, attention, emotion, prejudice, etc) some operating at the time of original event, during storage and still others operating at the time of recall. An organism without a capacity for memory is not able to profit from experience or training, to use association to predict what will be on the basis of what was.

DIFFERENT CONCEPTUALIZATIONS OF HUMAN MEMORY

Socrates thought memory as a black wax as whatever information is stored, it is imprinted on the wax, the moment the imprinting is removed, memory diminishes. Aristotle conceived of memory as a mirror that presents the objects required by the intellectual to it. According to him memory is initiated by perception and is a part of perception. According to British Associationism memory is composed of ideas that are contigous *i.e.,* ideas that follow each other. Herman Ebbinghaus (1885) wrote a book called "memory". During his time no systematic formulation of memory structure existed, no sophisticated apparatus was available and no data base of previous experimentation existed. Thus, his exploration of the unknown properties of memory was undertaken with little information to guide him. To negate the effect of any prior experiences he used the non-sense syllables. Forgetting was maximum at the initial intervals and decreased as the intervals increased. He used paired-associate technique. He also demonstrated the "serial-position effect." He found that with repetition of syllables series individual items associate with their immediate sequence and connection are also established between each item and several of those follow it. He talked about 'remote associations *i.e.,* the strength of association is inversely proportional to the distance b/w the items.

James was the one who differentiated between primary and secondary memory. Primary is the more immediate memory whereas secondary memory is more deep rooted. His secondary memory is somewhat similar to Freud's unconscious. He says that memory has two characteristics *i.e.,* it is permanent as well as transitory. These two systems were distinguished by Waugh and Norman in 1965. In this model, a verbal item enters primary memory and held by rehearsals or it may be forgotten. Due to rehearsal, item enter into secondary memory.

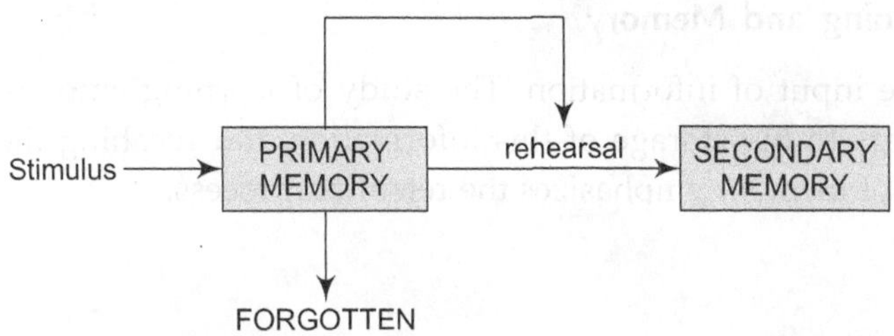

Model of Primary and Secondary Memory: Waugh and Norman (1975)

"Memory is a flexible, selective, changing process that our "remembrances of things past" are imperfect, distorted or just not recorded at all. And we think we remember events that never happened." E. F. Loftus (1980). Memory is seldom an accurate record of what was experienced because it is a subjective rather than an objective record. Memory depends upon encoders' interpretation of that event. This interpretation is in turn a result of encoders' perception of the world in terms of schemas, stereotypes, biases and assumptions. Moreover, this inference constructed on the basis of prior knowledge continue to influence the new information.—Loftus (1980). In analyzing memory, William Brewer and J. R. Pani (1983) have suggested that the contents of our memory can be categorized into *Personal Memories* consist of distinct episodes such as this morning's breakfast. When we remember such episodes, we can "see" the event taking place, and our mental images carry a sense of the past. *Generic memories,* include memories that are abstract and are not tied to any particular time or place; we do not remember where we learned them. They include memories that are primarily semantic/meaning-related, rather than being scenes. These memories also include perceptual memories of the way things look, sound or smell. *Skill memories* consists of cognitive skills, such as our ability to solve quadratic equations; motor skills etc.

Role of Memory

1. Memories help you define yourself
2. Connect with your present thoughts and actions to the roots of your past
3. Prepare for a meaningful future
4. They form a living record of what you have heard, read and experienced over the period of your life.
5. Memories blend past reality with expectation, fantasy and social desirability.

Difference b/w Human Memory and Computer Memory

Units of information are stored in brains. A brain uses graded and changing signals and processes many different kinds of information at the same time. A human has the ability to process different information at one time. This process is known as parallel processing. Brain's memory units are not as stable and unchanging as those of computer. Bits of information are stored in a computer's databank. A computer uses transistor, i.e., processes one information at a time responding to only two signals !(on) and 0 (off). A computer that processes one piece of information at a time is called a serial processor. A computer does not spontaneously add to or modify its stored memories.

Difference b/w Learning and Memory

Learning refers to the input of information. The study of learning emphasizes the acquisition process. Memory refers to the storage of this information and recalling the information when required while study of memory emphasizes the retention process.

Memory Theories

Broadbent's filter theory (1958)

Broadbent developed a theory of attention. He said that a lot of stimuli act collectively on the organism. Whatever information is received the relevant information moves on to the STM and the remaining is filtered out. He regarded mind as a communicatory channel which is the active processor and transmitter of information. He was the 1st psychologist to describe functions with a flow character. According to him cognition is a flow of information through the organism. Several arrows indicate people receiving more information than they can process. The selective filter blocks the unwanted input letting through only messages that merit full cognitive analysis. It can be variably tuned. According to this theory, a great deal of information can be stored in the sensory channels simultaneously but evacuating information from the sensory register is a laborious process that must be done serially, *i.e.,* one channel at a time. This had been confirmed by Cherry and Mowbray's findings. They found that subjects could apparently extract the meaning of only one story when two had been presented-one visually, the other aurally. In this case, the decrement in performance was produced by the selection filters inability to switch between the auditory and visual channels. This proves that focus of attention is determined by 3 components: a selective filter which led to a channel of limited capacity which in turn led to device detection.

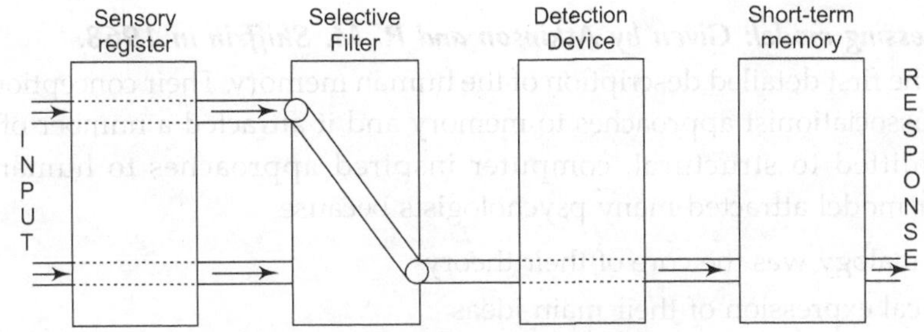

Broadbent Theory of Attention

Neisser worked in the area of artificial intelligence i.e., computer technology and software. He was concerned with the problem of recognition patterns/processes. He gave the concept of iconic memory which holds information for about 1/2 a second similar to Atkinsons and Shiffrin sensory register. He also gave the concept of active verbal memory which became the STM of Atkinson and Shiffrin. He also formed parallel processing in tasks involving visual search. In 1967 he formulated a view of attention that accommodated both the data driven phenomenon emphasized by Broadbend and the conceptually driven phenomena emphasized by Norman. His iconic memory and Broadbent buffer became the sensory register of Atkinson and Shiffrin. James primary memory and Broadbent's limited capacity store became STM of Atkinson and Shiffrin. James secondary memory became the LTM of Atkinson and Shiffrin. Sperling (1960): has conducted some of the classic studies in the area of sensory storage. These studies demonstrate that humans seem to have an extremely accurate and complete memory for visual stimulation although this memory's duration is brief. Moreover, he found that the way in which the stimuli were arranged on the tachistoscope slide didn't seem to have any effect on the subject's retrieval. Also the number of elements in the array didn't seem to produce any effect on retrieval. Finally, even when exposure time was increased dramatically, up to 5/10th of a sec. the number of elements retrieved stayed constant. This last finding indicates that the upperlimit of retrieved items was not imposed by any difficulty in seeing the items. Now, what was the nature of memory deficit? Was it one of capacity or one of duration? Sperling abandoned the whole report technique in which he had asked the subjects to retrieve as much as they could from the array. He substituted the partial report technique. The subjects were now required to report only certain elements of the preceding display. In this S's accuracy was good. Later on he argued that visual information is recognized, elaborated, rehearsed after the sensory storage. Sperling found that material in the sensory register is stored without any attempt at pattern recognition. He found that icons durability was strongly influenced by the adaptive state of the viewer's eye.

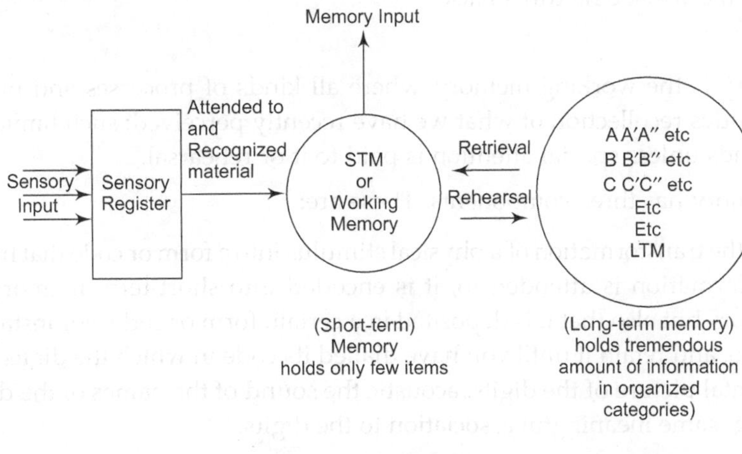

Information processing model: Given by Atkinson and R. M. Shiffrin in 1968.

This model was the first detailed description of the human memory. Their conception was a radical departure from associationist approaches to memory and it attracted a number of psychologists who were committed to structural, computer inspired approaches to human information processing. Their model attracted many psychologists because:

(a) computer analogy was the core of their theory
(b) mathematical expression of their main ideas
(c) application of the conceptual core to lab. Data of the verbal learning type.
(d) Atkinson and Shiffrin adopted a pre-theoretical view. They distinguished structural features from control processes. STM from LTM and sensory register. Their model used standard verbal learning techniques. They proposed that memory has hierarchy of levels in terms of three memory stores which they call sensory register, short-term store and long-term store. These stores are structurally distinct because they preserve information:
    (a) In different formats
    (b) For different durations
    (c) For different purposes
    (d) They loose information in different ways and
    (e) Have different anatomical bases.

Information processing approach there is a sensory memory, STM and LTM.

Sensory memory: preserves fleeting impressions of sensory stimuli—sights, sounds, smells and textures for only a second or two. There are three processes: Encoding: visual information is held in sensory memory in the form of an image. This image is a copy of the visual input and is called an iconic image. A similar phenomenon for the auditory system is known as echoic memory.

Storage: it accommodates up to at least 16 items. May be more at times. Visual input is held up to two secs. Auditory input is held up to five sec.

Information is lost due to decay and displacement by new information. If items are attended they may move to short-term memory. Sperling studies show that sensory register holds visual items (11 to 16) before it looses the information through decay.

Retrieval is possible. When stimulus is as long as there, then we can retrieve. For example, on station man hears the whistle he turns back.

Short-term memory

Short-term memory is the working memory, where all kinds of processes and problem solving takes place. It includes recollection of what we have recently perceived; such limited information lasts upto 20 seconds unless special attention is paid to it or rehearsal.

Short-term memory has three components. These are:

Encoding: refers to the transformation of a physical stimulus into a form or code that human memory accepts. When information is attended to, it is encoded into short-term memory. Information deposited in memory but also that it is deposited in a certain form or code. For instance, when you look up a phone no. and retain it until you have dialled its code in which the digits stored may be in visual form-mental picture of the digits, acoustic the sound of the names of the digits, semantic (based on meaning) same meaningful association to the digits.

Storage: refers to the retention of information that is encoded. Storage is the storehouse of consciousness. It has limited capacity. Ebbinghaus, was the one who decided to measure objectively. He reported that on an average people store seven items. Few store five and other can store upto nine items. (7+/-2)last for 20–30 seconds. Storage capacity of short-term memory can be increased by two ways.

(a) chunking

(b) rehearsal

Retrieval: from the STM has been studied experimentally by Sternberg. Retrieval requires a search of STM in which the items are examined one at a time.

Long-term memory

Long-term memory stores large amounts of information over a long period of time-days, months, years and even a lifetime. Items are stored sequentially according to their meanings perhaps many meanings for one item and numerous cross references to related material. Long-term memory by contrast is more like a set of file cabinets or library.

Encoding:

1. Information in LTM is episodic as well as semantic.
2. Organization of information in LTM is subjective as individual may organize the material to be remembered in his/her own way. This is known as subjective organization.
3. Information which is to be remembered may be meaningful but connections b/w them are not. In such a case, an individual may think up a real or artificial link b/w the items.
4. Coding by meaning and forming a visual image also helps in other forms of coding of verbal material in LTM.

Storage: storage capacity of LTM is unlimited. Loss of information may be due to inadequate encoding, time decay, interference, failure to consolidate, motivated forgetting, retrieval failure.

Information stored is organized: the tip of the tongue phenomenon supports the fact that information in LTM is organized.

Retrieval: search in LTM is not random. While retrieving the information a search is generated in the appropriate part of memory after which the item is located, or contacted, recognized and recalled. Item may be there in LTM but failure to recall the item due to inappropriate retrieval strategy or interference-forgetting occurs.

Methods of retrieval: Recall

1. Recall means reproducing the information to which you were previously exposed.
2. If a police asked a victim to describe from memory, the persons distinguishing features. Did you notice anything unusual about the attacker.
3. Recall questions usually give fewer cues and less specific ones.
4. For recall you must reconstruct from memory something that is not in the present environment and then describe it.

Recognition:

1. Recognition means realizing that a certain stimulus event is one you have seen or heard before.

2. If a police asked a victim to describe criminal, he/she could be shown photos one at a time to identify the suspect.
3. Recognition questions give more cues and more specific ones.
4. For recognition you need to simply match a remembered stimulus against a present perception.

Atkinson and Shiffrin drew a Difference b/w the three memory stores in terms:

(a) Duration of information held: At sensory register is less than 1 second, as long as information attended to and for 15-30 second if not attended to whereas for LTM it is indefinitely and often permanent.

(b) Form of information: visual and auditory in case of sensory register, Auditory verbal-linguistic (A VL) is STM store and visual, AVL, olfactory, temporal in LTM.

(c) Source of information: is the senses in case of sensory register.

(d) Information capacity: unknown but large for sensory register; small for STM and unlimited for LTM.

(e) Forgetting: due to decay, erasure by overwriting in sensory register, decay in STM and decay and interference of various sorts in LTM.

(f) Function: only STM allows for conscious manipulations of information.

Criticisms of information processing approach

Concept of chunks has been postulated to account for variable data in STM. This involves basic consumption that STM is very flexible and can accept the variety of codes from simple physical features to complex semantic ones. This notion is against the basic postulate of multi-store model.

1. **Coding:** It was generally considered that only the long-term store could maintain semantic information *i.e.,* meaning based codes. The short-term store accepts only acoustically coded-information. However, experiments by Shulman (1970,72) suggested that semantic codes could also be held in short-term store.
2. **Capacity:** The sensory register is considered to have capacity, long-terms capacity to store information is unlimited but the capacity for STM is thought to be quite small. This is another assumption of the multistore models. It explains forgetting during input. Experimental estimates of the short-term stores capacity turned out to be highly variable. Depending on the kind of material used, the short-term store seemed capable of maintaining anywhere from two to 20 words. Craik and Lockhart (1972). Two words are implausible. This shows that capacity of STM store varies:-Further two theoretical questions about the capacity limit of the STM were never satisfactorily resolved. (Peterson, 1977). First, the mechanism by which the store loses information was never clearly established. Some argued that it is by displacement, others said that loss is due to a combination of displacement and decay but the number of units that could be maintained by rehearsal was strictly limited. Second, whether the capacity limits stemmed from an inability to hold more than a fixed number of items at one time, or an inability to rehearse more than a fixed number of items during any given time.-(craik and Lockhart 1972)
3. **Forgetting Functions:** Early experiments that supported the forgetting functions of multistore model showed that—information is lost from sensory register in a second or less and from STM in five second without rehearsal. The LTM was supposed to hold information for indefinite period of time. But, the subsequent experiments yield widely different estimates

for Icon and STM store. For Icon, Posner (1969) estimated up to 1.5 sec. Murdock (1971) estimated 6 sec. Philips and Baddeley (1971) 10 sec for STM store, Peterson and Peterson reported 15–20 sec. for complete loss of information from STM without rehearsal. Craik and Lockhart reported beyond 20 second. These results disqualified the assumption of multi-store model!

5. Atkinson and Shiffrin postulated an unconscious mechanism for the transfer of information from the short to long-term store. They did not specify the character of this mechanism but they did specify one of its results. The longer the information remains in the short-term store the more strongly it is presented in the long-term store.
6. **Conceptual problems with multistore models:** Atkinson-Shiffrin model is criticized largely because of the following reasons:
   (a) the model do not account for human activities that have meaning at their core
   (b) some cognitive Psychologists believe that the model is insufficient in principle while others believe that extending them is impractical and hopelessly complex.

Alternate models of memory as multistore model by Atkinson and Shiffrin

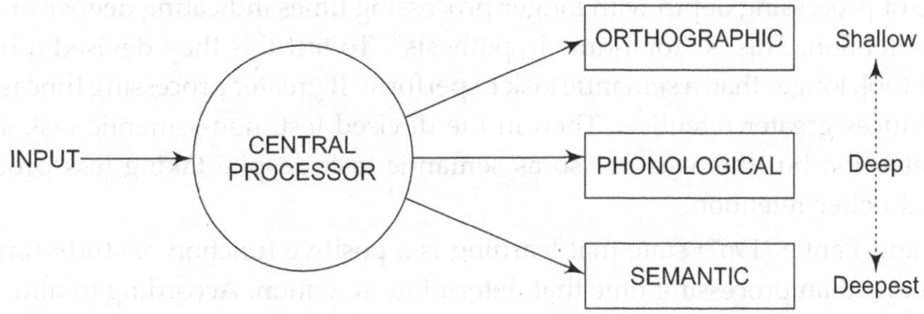

According to Craik and Lockhart, memory depends upon the nature of the code and not on the properties of memory stores. Different codes have different permanence. Life of a given code can be lengthened by "receiving" or updating it. According to Craik updating does not change the level of processing because that is fixed by the nature of the input code. Nor does the recirculation improve later memory of the input—as rehearsal was said by multistore models. Recirculation simply extends the life of a code while it is updated.

For example: Repetition of a telephone number while waiting to dial it. When the no. is read the perceptual analysis extract an acoustic code that does not persist unless it is updated.

Postulates Craik and Lockhart's level of processing are based on similar distinction between STM and LTM as in case of multi-store models. But Craik and Lockhart gave two kinds of memory primary and secondary. Primary is responsible for whatever is being actively processed. Secondary memory contains records of past-analysis and comprises what the person knows without thinking about it.

Features of LOP: Craik and Lockhart proposed that processing of a stimulus could be undertaken at a number of different levels. They proposed three encoding dimensions:

(a) Orthographic
(b) Phonological
(c) Semantic

They envisaged these encoding dimensions on a continuum stretching from "shallow" to "deep" levels. Shallow Deep Deepest (orthography) (phonology) (semantic)

Orthographic processing produces the poorest level of memory, then phonological processing. Semantic Processing produces the greatest level of retention.

They proposed that processing of a stimulus is under the control of a central processor. Central processor is a system with limited but flexible capacity that dealt with the processing of new information, the deeper the level , the better the retention, because retention of a stimulus depends on the way central processor deployed during learning.

Criticisms of LOP approach

Through Craik and Tulving (1975) never claimed LOP as a theory as they always called it a 'framework for memory research'. But the other theorists who treated it as a theory criticized LOP as a theory of memory.

- Craik and Tulving (1975) proposed that semantic orienting tasks always took longer to perform than non-semantic ones. They reasoned that processing time is an effective independent measure of processing depth with longer processing times indicating deeper processing and greater retention. This is "total-time hypothesis". To test this they devised a non-semantic task that took longer than a semantic task to perform. If greater processing time is the variable that produces greater retention. Then in the devised test, non-semantic task should show better retention but this was not so as semantic task despite taking less processing time produced better retention.
- Cooper and Pantle (1967) state that learning is a positive function of study time. There are other factors than processing time that determines retention. According to him, relationship between learning and memory is determined by more than just how long we spend attending to the stimulus out of which qualitative differences in the way information is encoded could be one.
- Craik and Lockhart did explain that performance is measured by recall. But could not explain how to measure performance in recognition memory. Craik and Lockhart's framework is based on central assumption that information is processed by the attention primary memory system through a hierarchy of levels beginning with physical features and moving in case of words through phonemic features to a semantic level.
- But Wingrad (1972) said that such a hierarchical processing takes place in a computer and not in the human memory. He said three component programmes—one for analyzing syntax, one for semantics and third for reasoning. All these three components interacts and not operate in series. As by doing this a powerful language analysis is produced and humans are capable of doing this.

Conclusion: Craik and Lockhart did not make levels of processing into a concrete theory. Rather they advanced it as a conceptual orientation that emphasizes the role of memory processes instead of multistore model.

FORGETTING

Forgetting refers to the apparent loss of information already encoded and stored in LTM.

Factors Causing Forgetting

Theory of storage failure

Information lost from storage due to displacement by subsequent information or to decay with time or due to inappropriate encoding.

Interference

If we associate different items to the same cue when we try to use that cue to retrieve one of the items the other items will come to mind and interfere with our recovery of the target.

Decay theory of forgetting

The associative approach has explained forgetting in terms of the decay theory. According to associative approach memories are based on associations between ideas. According to this theory—forgetting occurs when the passage of time weakens the bond. It assumes that learning leaves a trace in the brain which gets decayed or faded with time and disappears after prolonged disuse. And such a fading or decay is believed to occur as a normal metabolic process of the brain.

Criticisms

Retrieval system may get weakened

(a) due to old age. Although information is there, but it takes time for them to retrieve.
(b) due to shocks
(c) due to accidents
(d) transfer of information from STM to LTM pathways get disrupted which may lead to retrieval.

Theory of cue dependent forgetting

This theory puts forth the view that forgetting is caused by failure to retrieve information from storage due to inadequate memory cues. For example: you are trying to recall a person whom you met at a party whose name or face you do not remember. Just then a friend describes the dress of this person. You realize that you are now able to recall this person. Dress-retrieval cue.

Displacement

If attention is paid to the information it is transmitted to short-term store. The STM has a limited capacity. Thus, if too much information is pushed out. Thus there is no retention of the information pushed or displaced. Also if the information in STM is not rehearsed then that information too may be lost.

Theory of motivated forgetting

Freud developed this theory based on the observation of his patients. Freud used this term 'repression' to refer to the tendency of individuals to avoid remembering anything associated with fear or unpleasantness. The memories that arouse pain, discomfort or anxiety are likely to be blocked or repressed. For example: soldiers returning from battlefield suffer from amnesia—loss of memory—related to their suffering and combat experiences. Moreover, shameful experiences are often forgotten.

Other factors which hinder retrieval are:

(a) negative emotions hinder retrieval
(b) emotional context situations

For example: if you learn a material in an unpleasant mood retrieval will be better if you were asked to retrieve in an unhappy mood.

(c) For unemotional situations retrieval is not as better as in emotional situations. For example: you may forget a movie which you saw in a theatre but if a fire breaks out while you are in a theatre, you will describe the setting over and over to friends, thereby rehearsing and organizing it.

CURRENT STATE OF RESEARCH ON MEMORY

Different research trends have emerged after multistore model and LOP approach. These are: Some are attempting to develop alternate theories. Some are attempting to develop and extend the three store model concepts. Most of the researchers are dealing with specific questions only. As they are trying to explain reliable information without reference to any broad integrative theory.

A large group of studies concern the free recall of unrelated list of words and others compare recognition and recall memory. Some are trying to improve multistore models. Some assumptions of multistore and LOP retained are: that information enters the memory systems through some sensory "buffer"; STM has a limited capacity and existence of iconic and echoic storage is not discounted.

MNEMONICS

The aids to improve our memory are called as mnemonics. Few popular ways of improving memory are:

- Learning the material in one emotional state and recalling it in the same emotional state.
- Learning of material associated with the place of visit or happening. Recall is better when the person visits that place.
- Learning the material with some rhyming such as one for bun, two for shoe.

REFLECT YOURSELF

1. Write a short note on mnemonics.
2. Elucidate upon current state of research in memory.
3. Delineate the different approaches to study memory.
4. Write a short note on information processing approach.

7

THINKING

TOPICS COVERED IN THIS CHAPTER
• Introduction • Role of Images and Language in Thinking • Defining a Concept • Define Problem Solving and State Nature and Strategies of Problem Solving • Prototype • Creative Thinking

INTRODUCTION

Mr. Lamuel prepares for the lecture, got up late in the morning and has to rush or else he will miss the train at subway. For all such problems, how he reacts will not only show his thinking skills but also sets him apart from others who also face similar problems in their life. What are these mental operations? What are these skills which differentiates from one individual to another. Let's take a look. Thinking is an important cognitive process involving the cognitive rearrangement of information from the environment and of symbols stored in the memory, leading to the sense of personal identity, providing context for our perception and helping in representing our experiences.

Various Approaches to Define the Concept of Thinking

Thinking occurs almost all the time and yet it is difficult to define it. So various approaches are made in order to define thinking. These are discussed below:

1. According to John B. Watson thinking is considered as a case of subvocal speech in which an external stimulus produced a behavioural response.
2. Another approach views thinking as information processing that occurs between a stimulus event and the response to the event. E.g. sight of the ad of a bike is a stimulus event and

decision of buying is response. This means that thinking mediates between the stimulus situation and the response.

3. In the last decades, the study of thinking has shifted towards a cognitive perspective. Thus, cognitive process refers to the processes involved in the formation and utilization of symbols and concepts associated with thinking, reasoning, problem solving, creativity and decision-making,etc. Hence, this approach mentions cognitive modalities in terms of visual-auditory, sensory-motor or verbal.

ROLE OF IMAGES AND LANGUAGE IN THINKING

The role of images and language in thinking is discussed below:

Images are pictures in brain. They are abstractions of certain features of previous experiences. Images used in thinking are usually incomplete pictures. They involve memory of a percept without any stimulus being present. They occur in every sense modality, in terms of sensory motor or verbal, visual-auditory. Since images are abstractions of information stored in memory may be used in problem solving. People differ in the extent to which they tend to imagine things.

Similarly language also plays an important role in thinking process. Language and thought are interdependent. According to B.L. Whorf, language people use to determine and shapes their experience and thought process. According to his theory of linguistic relativity, but according to Watson thinking is a subvocal speech or a kind of silent talk. Since language is a late invention so language is a tool for thinking and processes of thinking, primarily determine the nature of language.

DEFINING A CONCEPT

Describe the types of concept with examples

- Concept are important language symbols used in thinking. The human ability to form concept enables us to classify things into categories.
- A concept is a symbolic construction that represents some common and general features of many objects and things. They help us to classify and organize our world of experience and improve our ability to adapt to environment. We classify people, objects, events or people's behaviour, it means that one has developed a concept about them. Thus, concept refers to making the same response to a group of objects having similar characteristics. A concept is a category or class of objects or events grouped or combined on the basis of a rule which specifies the relevant feature or features.

Types of Concepts

Simple and complex. Complex split into three —conjunctive, disjunctive and relational. Simple concepts are defined by a single feature or property, e.g. red, blue, yellow and green. Complex concepts are defined by several common properties. E.g. red square. Conjunctive concept represents two or more features of an object at a time.

E.g. red square. A disjunctive concept represents anyone of the several attributes of an item e.g. either red or square.

Relational concepts denote relationships between features of objects or events. E.g. a house with more doors than windows. Other examples are—smaller than, taller than.

Process of Concept Attainment

Generalization and discrimination are two processes which operate while attaining the concepts. For concept attainment we must identify the relevant and the irrelevant attributes of an object or event. For this it requires the ability to detect the rule governing the relevant attributes. Thus, concept attainment involves the two-fold activities *i.e.,* Attribute discovery and rule discovery. The process of concept attainment is discussed below: a subject is trying to attain the concept in an experimental situation. He/she does not behave randomly and uses hypothetical testing. he/she is presented with a number of examples and non-examples of the concept. In this situation subject tries to identify the relevant and the irrelevant attributes of the object or event. He/she forms hypothesis and report. If it belongs to the concept then the S is told by the E that his/her response is right. I fit is not then his/her response is reported wrong. From the feedback generalizations and discrimination process take place, due to which S develops the ability to detect the rule governing relevant attributes.

DEFINE PROBLEM SOLVING AND STATE NATURE AND STRATEGIES OF PROBLEM SOLVING

- Problem solving is an important cognitive activity. It is the process of moving from the given state to the goal state of a problem. The nature of problem solving is discussed below:
- It involves situations in which something is blocking the successful completion of a task A. There are three aspects of a problem.

(a) Original state: is a situation at the beginning when one encounters the problem. (b) Goal state: is a situation which is reached when the problem is solved. (c) Rule: are those procedural details which must be followed or taken in account while proceeding from the original state to the goal state.

Problem solving emerges out of conceptual behaviour. Some problem are simple, clear and some are complex. Long and complex procedure is to be followed for the solution of a complex natured problem.

Good Strategies Help in Problem Solving by Minimizing the Processing and Remembering of Information

These are listed below:

1. Algorithms: are procedures or rules that guarantee the solution to a given problem. Algorithms lead to mechanical solutions. They take time, lengthy but specific procedure is followed.
2. Heuristics: are short-cut rules of thumb that often lead to quick solutions. These are simpler and less demanding strategies as compared to algorithms, but they may or may not yield situations. They are based on past experiences and involve reasoning. They are helpful in real life situations.

3. Means end analysis: this approach involves the division of problem into a number of subproblems each of which is a little closer to the desired goal thus reducing or eliminating the differences between the current state of the problem and the solution. It is useful in solving chess problem, in programming computers as well as day to day problems.
4. Backward search: the problem is broken into the smaller sections which are easier to manage. The problem solver starts at the goal state and works backwards to the given initial state. This strategy is useful in case of those problems where the goal has more information than the given problem and the nature of the problem is such that the operations can be conducted in a forward and backward direction. E.g. Normally this method is followed in public gatherings like republic day or marriage.

Factors Affecting Problem Solving

1. Mental set: set refers to the way of perceiving certain structure or situation. Mental set may create hindrance in problem solving when the problem requires new solutions, new rules or new applications of previous experience.
2. Rigidity: a kin to mental set or perceptual set there is a kind of response set which involves continuing to use a response that worked in other situation. This is rigidity which we call habits in a layman's language. E.g. person working on computer.
3. Functional fixedness: it is the set in our mind that one particular object functions in that very manner. When the function of a particular object is fixed or determined by its use in a particular way just before the problem is presented it is called functional fixedness. It blocks the thinking process when we are faced with problems that require novel and insightful solutions.
4. Well defined and ill defined problems: In well defined problems-goals are well-defined, the information necessary to solve the problem is specified precisely in the statement of the problem. In ill-defined problem-the goals are vague, the relevant information is not specified.
5. Anxiety: in some problems goals give rise to conflicting motives and values, which are likely to hinder problem solving, conflicts and frustrations give rise to anxiety.
6. Attention span: limitations of working memory may restrict the capacity to work with more than a few problem solving operations at a time.
7. Incubation: refers to the increase in the likelihood of solving a problem that results from delaying, rest or withdrawal for some time from the problem under consideration.
8. Brainstorming: it is a process by which individuals are encouraged to produce solutions of problems in the group. In general larger number of solution which may be of good quality are produced by brainstorming. This strategy overcomes the problem of fixedness which hinders problem solving.

PROTOTYPE

The particular example of the concept that readily comes to mind is called the prototype of that concept. It has been found that categories based on prototypes are acquired quickly and prototypes serve as reference points. The easiest and the first example which come into our mind without thinking at all is called prototype of that concept. It has been found that this example has maximum characteristics of the concept and is truly representative of that concept.

CREATIVE THINKING

Creative Thinking Skills

Unconventional. Uninhibited. Risk-taker. Always looks for new patterns and new combinations. Inventive. Extremely curious. Driven. Visionary: Intuitive Rather individualistic.

Barriers to Creativity

The diagram shows barriers to creativity. Lack of self-motivation is a barrier to creativity because if the individual is having complexes and low selfesteem which further develops into low self confidence resulting in negative attitude leads hinders in creative task. If the country's economy is experiencing a slump resulting in stress level among the nationals, the educational system is also at stake where even the brilliant minds experience sacking. Corporate culture, say that of Indian bureaucracy where red-tapism has eaten up the creativity. This further gets support from our country's economical and political situation. Further if the family background believes in handing over their culture to the offsprings then that also hinder creativity because it may lead too many rules and formalization which may be a misfit in contemporary scenario.

Types of Creative Thinking Styles

Brain storming

Brainstorming is a technique which is widely used when we need the group to get into decision-making process. In such a process, every group member gives out a possible solution and at the end, one gets a wide range of solutions.

Mind mapping

Hierarchal Breakdown and Exploration: in this technique, the potential problem is broken down into a stepwise fashion and possible solutions are explored. Hence reaching out for the solution to the original problem.

Absence thinking

Thinking About What is Not There: in this problem solving technique, one takes out into account of those aspects of problem which is not reflected in the original problem. Thus, the problem solver has to think about possible\solutions to those of the problem which are invisible in a given state.

Talk streaming

Talking, Talking and Talking Until Unblocking: it is the technique, which puts the creative thinker to talk about the possible solutions till he gets hang of the solution to the problem.

Attribute listing

Listing Attributes of Objects and then Challenging them: it is a situation where the problem solver lists the attributes of the problem situation and challenge them with each solution that they enlist.

Assumption busting

Challenging Unconscious Assumptions: it is a situation, where the problem solver addresses the unconscious assumptions on which the problem is based and potential answers are directed toward solving the problem.

Visioning

Creating a Motivating View of the Future: it is a situation where the problem solver delineates a vision for himself and tries to formulate solutions for the motivating tomorrow.

Wishing

Stating Ideas as Wishes to Expand Thinking: when the problem solver has a vision with a mission before himself. He thus, tries to expand the horizon of his success by stating ideas in order to expand his thinking process.

Pausing

- **Think More Deeply for a Minute:** it is a situation, where the problem solver brings out a pause, where he thinks more deeply for a minute.

  Taking a Break

- **When Creativity is Fading:** it is a situation when the problem solver takes a break when creativity begins to fade. Like in all insightful situations, where a break into getting solutions brings out a solution by breaking a chain of thoughts!

  Edward de Bono's

  Six Thinking Hats

  Provides a framework for thinking:

  Facts—what do we already know?

  Emotions—how do we feel about this?

  Caution, bad points

  Optimism, good points

  Creativity, new ideas

  Process—thinking about thinking

Stages in Creative Thinking

1. Preparation: the thinker formulates the problem and collects facts and materials considered necessary for the new solution.
2. Incubation: the thinker either deliberately or involuntarily'tums away from it.
3. Illumination: 'aha' insight experience occurs.
4. Evaluation: the apparent solution is tested to see if it satisfactorily solves the problem.
5. Revision: is reached. Steps taken so far.

Characteristics of Creative Thinkers

1. They prefer complexity and some degree of apparent imbalance in phenomena.
2. They are more complex psychodynamically and have greater personal scope.
3. They are more independent in their judgements.
4. They are more self-assertive and dominant.
5. They reject suppression as a mechanism for the control of impulse.

REFLECT YOURSELF

1. Write short note on creative thinking.
2. What is the meaning of prototype?
3. Discuss the stages in problem solving.

8

PERSONALITY

TOPICS COVERED IN THIS CHAPTER

- Introduction
- Types of Personality Theories
- Alteration in Personality
- Psychological Assessments of Personality

INTRODUCTION

A brief definition would be that personality is made up of the characteristic patterns of thoughts, feelings and behaviours that make a person unique. In addition to this, personality arises from within the individual and remains fairly consistent throughout life.

Some of the fundamental characteristics of personality include:

- **Consistency:** There is generally a recognizable order and regularity to behaviours. Essentially, people act in the same ways or similar ways in a variety of situations.
- **Psychological and physiological:** Personality is a psychological construct, but research suggests that it is also influenced by biological processes and needs.
- **Impact behaviours and actions:** Personality does not just influence how we move and respond in our environment; it also *causes* us to act in certain ways.
- **Multiple expressions:** Personality is displayed in more than just behaviour. It can also be seen in out thoughts, feelings, close relationships and other social interactions.

In other words, "Personality" can be defined as a dynamic and organized set of characteristics possessed by a person that uniquely influences his or her cognitions, motivations, and behaviours in various situations."

Definition of Personality

The term 'personality' is derived from the Latin word "persona" which means mask. The Greek actors used masks to hide their identity on stage. A number of theorists attempted to describe and define personality. R.S. Woodworth defined personality as the "quality of the individual's total behaviour". The most widely accepted definition is the one given by Gordon Allport. According to G. Allport, "personality is the dynamic organization within the individual, of those psychophysical systems that determine his characteristic behaviour and thought". The key concepts are explained below:

- Dynamic: refers to the constantly evolving, changing nature of personality. As the individual grows, his physical and physiological aspects develop and change from time to time and situation to situation.
- Organization: emphasizes that different systems of personality have special relation to the whole. It points out that personality is not just a sum total of traits added to one another, rather different traits or manifest aspects of the personality pattern are held together and influenced by a central core which is commonly known as 'self'.
- Psychophysical systems: is composed of habits, attitudes, emotional states, motives and beliefs which are psychological in nature but they have a physical basis in the individual's neural, glandular or general body states which constitute potentials for activity.
- Determine: emphasizes the motivational role of the psychophysical systems. Once an attitude, belief or some element of psychophysical system has been aroused by a stimulus either from the environment or within the individual it provokes adjustive and expressive acts which are characteristic forms of expressions of that particular individual.
- Characteristic: refers to the distinctiveness or uniqueness of the person's behaviour as an expression of his own psychophysical system.
- Behaviour and thought: ideas and activities which are the expressions of the personality directed towards the specific goal, enable the individual to adjust to his environment.

There are a number of different theories about how personality develops. Different schools of thought in psychology influence many of these theories. Some of these major perspectives on personality include:

TYPES OF PERSONALITY THEORIES

Psychodynamic Theory

Psychoanalytic theory of personality is founded by Sigmund Freud, and emphasizes the influence of the unconscious on personality. According to Freud we are motivated to satisfy instinctual needs (sexual)—libidinous energy. Unconscious conflicts are forcibly kept from awareness; this influences our behaviour. Past events shape subsequent behaviour. Psychologists sharing this approach attempted to identify deep psychological forces which are responsible for development, maintenance, and change of personality. Some called them as instincts and others claimed it to be needs that interact with the environment to produce the manifested personality. He made the arbitrary division of mind and called them the 'Conscious', the 'Preconscious' and the 'Unconscious'. Out of three , the unconscious was considered as the main principle behind human motivation. Everything you are aware of at a given moment. Preconscious mind-material that is unconscious, but can be easily brought into awareness. Moves back and forth easily between conscious and unconscious. Material that can easily be brought into awareness.

Unconscious mind—is completely outside of our awareness (could produce anxiety if made conscious). Holds repressed memories and emotions and the id's instinctual drives

Among the most basic notions are instinctual tendencies which account for human behaviour. The 'Eros' or the life instinct includes all behaviour connected with preservation, perpetuation and procreation of human life. The 'Thanatos' or the death instinct is connected with destruction of life.

1. **Eros**–The "life" instinct. Motivates us to survive.
2. **Thanatos**—Death wish. From moment of birth we are striving towards our death.

His concepts , the 'Id', the 'Ego' and the 'Superego' described three aspects of personality.

1. **Id**–unconscious impulses that want to be gratified, without regard to potential punishment. Is source of psychic energy **(libido).** Innate biological instincts and urges; selfserving and irrational. Totally unconscious. Works on **Pleasure Principle:** Wishes to have its desires (pleasurable) satisfied NOW, without waiting and regardless of the consequences.
2. **Ego (primarily conscious)**–tries to satisfy id impulses while minimizing punishment and guilt. Executive; directs id energies. Partially conscious and partially unconscious. Works on **Reality Principle:** Delays action until it is practical and/or appropriate.
3. **Superego**–the "moral" center of our personality which tells us right from wrong (somewhat conscious). Judge or censor for thoughts and actions of the ego Superego comes from our parents or caregivers; guilt comes from the superego Sigmund Freud.

Sigmund freud

Is a **stage theory**—Assumes one must pass each stage successfully to move on.

To release this tension, we externalize our aggression (act out toward others). Personality Development Freud argued that personality development is result of conflicts we resolve in childhood. We learn to satisfy id impulses while handling societal pressures.

Psychosexual stages of personality development

Oral stage: Ages 0-1. Most of infant's pleasure comes from stimulation of the mouth. Needs' to be gratified orally (sucking, chewing, biting). If a child is overfed or frustrated, oral traits will develop.

Fixations create oral–aggressive adults who like to argue and exploit others.

Erogenous zone: mouth (oral) anal stage: Ages 1–3. Attention turns to process of elimination. needs met—through elimination of waste. Either retaining or expelling feces. Child can gain approval or express aggression by letting go or holding on. Ego develops. Harsh or lenient toilet training can make a child either:

Anal retentive: Stubborn, stingy, orderly, and compulsively clean

Anal Expulsive: Disorderly, messy, destructive, or cruel

Erogenous zone: Anus phallic stage: Ages 3–6. needs met through genital stimulation (self-stimulation).Child now notices and is physically attracted to opposite sex parent. Can lead to:

Oedipus conflict: For boys only. Boy feels rivalry with his father for his mother's affection. Boy may feel threatened by father (castration anxiety). To resolve, boy must *identify* with his father (i.e., become more like him and adopt his heterosexual beliefs).

Electra conflict: Girl loves her father and competes with her mother. Girl identifies with her mother more slowly because she already feels castrated.

Erogenous Zone: Phallus

- **Latency:** Ages 6-Puberty. Psychosexual development is dormant. Same sex friendships and play occur here.
- **Genital Stage:** Puberty-on. Realization of full adult sexuality occurs here; sexual urges reawaken. Needs met through intercourse.

We become fixated at that stage and don't move on to the next stage. The concerns of that stage continue to dominate adult personality.

Handling anxiety

Freud argued we need to reduce the anxiety associated with unpleasant thoughts. To do this, we reject unpleasant thoughts from the conscious mind and force them into the unconscious mind. The "ego" employs "defense mechanisms" to regulate anxieties.

Cause of Anxiety Ego is always caught in the middle of battles between superego's desires for moral behaviour and the id's desires for immediate gratification. **Neurotic Anxiety:** Caused by id impulses that the ego can barely control. **Moral Anxiety:** Comes from threats of punishment from the superego.

Defense mechanism: a process used by the ego to distort reality and protect a person from anxiety.

Repression: the suppression of unpleasant thoughts. We push unpleasant thoughts into unconscious so that we can't access them. E.g., a child who is molested, may suppress the traumatic event so that he/she has no memory for the event.

Denial—refusing to believe something unpleasant has occurred. We refuse to accept horrible news, even with evidence to the contrary. E.g., you hear a friend has died and can't believe it's true.

Rationalization—we justify the actions or events that have happened. E.g. a student who decides to forgo studying for an exam the night before and goes out with friends.

Displacement—you take out your anger and frustration on a person or object not the actual target of your anger. E.g., After being grilled by your boss, you go home and yell at your partner or the dog/cat.

Projection—You attribute your negative characteristics to another person. When people project their own faults onto others, they generally do not deny that they themselves possess those faults. E.g., Your partner tells you how selfish you are, when they are in fact selfish.

Reaction Formation—acting the opposite of how you feel. You do the opposite of how you feel to defend your own doubts. E.g., A person who doubts his faith may act like a religious zealot to defend his religion.

Sublimation—the transformation of an unacceptable impulse into an acceptable behaviour. E.g., Aggressive impulses are transformed into the urge to engage in competitive sports. Most desirable way of dealing with unacceptable id impulses.

Undoing (atonement)—undoing is designed to negate or annul some disapproved thought, impulse or act. e.g., it is as if the individual has spelled a word wrong and used an eraser to clear the paper and start over. Apologizing for wrongs committed against others, penance, repentance, and undergoing punishment are all forms or undoing.

Emotional insulation—here the individual reduces his degree of emotional involvement in situations that might prove disappointing or hurtful. e.g., the student who is looking forward to a date with a very attractive girl may not let himself get too excited or enthusiastic for fear that something will happen to prevent it or that she will not like him such reactions will be expressed in common saying that "I didn't dare to even hope".

Sympathism and acting out—in the former the individual strives to gain the sympathy of others by telling about his "tough breaks", illnesses, and other difficulties. In this way his feelings of self worth are bolstered , despite his failures , by the expressions of concern and sympathy of others who realize how difficult it must be for one who is in illhealth or has had such bad luck. Acting out is a mechanism in which the individual reduces the anxiety aroused by forbidden desires by actually permitting their expressions. Thus rather than trying to repress immoral sexual or hostile urges which are anxiety arousing , he simply engages in the behaviour.

Criticisms of freud's theory

1. Freud had no scientific data to support his theories.
2. Freud's theories (unconscious, libido, etc.) cannot be observed.
3. Observations not representative of population. Pros of Freud's theory
   (a) Argued that **childhood experiences** are important in personality development.
   (b) Information outside of awareness **does influence us.**
   (c) Defense mechanisms—good descriptions of some of our behaviours.

Type Theory

These theories suggested that there are a limited number of "personality types" which are related to biological influences.

Carl Jung

A Swiss psychiatrist, Carl Jung who was a Freudian disciple, believed that we are one of two personality types:

Introvert

Shy, self-centered person whose attention is focused inward

Extrovert

Bold, outgoing person whose attention is directed outward

Hans eysenck

English psychologist, believed that there are three fundamental factors in personality:

Introversion versus Extroversion

Emotionally Stable versus Unstable (neurotic)

Impulse Control versus Psychotic

The first two factors create four combinations, related to the four basic temperaments recognized by ancient Greeks: **Melancholic** (introverted+unstable): sad, gloomy **Choleric** (extroverted+ unstable): hot-tempered, irritable **Phlegmatic** (introverted+stable): sluggish, calm **Sanguine** (extroverted+stable): cheerful, hopeful.

Trait Theory

Trait Theory viewed personality as the result of internal characteristics that are genetically based. According to the *Diagnostic and Statistical Manual* of the American Psychiatric. Association, personality traits are "enduring patterns of perceiving, relating to, and thinking about the environment and oneself that are exhibited in a widerange of social and personal contexts." Theorists generally assume (a) traits are relatively stable over time, (b) traits differ among individuals (e.g., some people are outgoing while others are reserved), and (c) traits influence behaviour.

Raymond cattell

From Devon, England, believed that there were two basic categories of traits:

Surface traits

Features that make up the visible areas of personality.

Source traits

Underlying characteristics of a personality. Cattell also constructed the *16PF,* a personality test identifying 16 personality factors (source traits and five "secondary factors."

Evaluation of trait theories

- Are traits as pervasive as trait theories claim? Is someone shy always or does it depend on the situation?
- Are traits as enduring and unchangeable as trait theories claim? Can we change our traits? If so, how easily? ·
- Are traits affected by social and cultural upbringing? Or are our personalities formed at birth and unchanging thereafter?

Difference between trait and type theory of personality is discussed as follows. Trait theorists centered their research around common, unique, cardinal and 16 factor approach. *Central traits* are basic to an individual's personality, while *secondary traits* are more peripheral.

Common traits are those recognized within a culture and thus may vary from culture to culture. *Cardinal traits* are those by which an individual may be strongly recognized. Type could be based upon temperament and body built.

Difference between Allport and Cattell's approach to personality is discussed as follows. The pioneering American psychologist Gordon Allport (1937) described two major ways to study personality: the nomothetic and the idiographic. *Nomothetic psychology* seeks general laws that can be applied to many different people, such as the principle of self-actualization, or the trait of extraversion. *Idiographic psychology* is an attempt to understand the unique aspects of a particular individual. Gordon Allport and R. Cattell have developed their theory of personality around the central concept called traits. Trait is defined as the unique organization of relatively enduring psychological characteristic possessed by an individual , revealed by his interaction. Cattell used statistical technique called factor analysis to study various dimensions of personality. This technique reveals that how traits are correlated and identified important cluster of linked traits. He identified 16 source traits that underlie differences among individuals. While Allport did not use any statistical technique to identify traits. Instead he classified traits into common traits which are found in all individuals under nomothetic approach and unique traits which are characteristic of a specific individual's personality under his idiographic approach. Allport also noted that few people are dominated by a single trait which he named as cardinal trait. Eg. Alexander the great-cardinal trait is ambition.

Social-Cognitive Theories

Bandura's theory

Alben Bandura also saw problems with the traditional behaviourist's view of personality. He argued that some behaviours that we exhibit are strictly human behaviours and that studying animals can never give us a compete understanding of human nature. The one major difference between human and lower animals, according to Bandura, is our advanced ability to process information.

His theory, known now as Social-Cognitive Theory, states that two aspects of human nature determine behaviour: internal and external. He called these reciprocal determinants of behaviour because they act together and cannot be separated. Since the outcome of our internal and external determinants can also influence future behaviour, **Self-system:** the set of cognitive processes by which a person observes, evaluates, and regulates his/her behaviour. Bandura proposed that what we think of as personality is a product of this self-system. Children observe behaviour of models (such as parents) in their social environment. Particularly if they are reinforced, children will imitate these behaviours, incorporating them into personality. Bandura also proposed that people observe their own behaviour and judge its effectiveness. **Self-efficacy:** a judgment of one's effectiveness in dealing with particular situations.

Julian rotter

Rotter's Theory of Locus of Control

Julian Rotter: American psychologist, began as a Freudian! His personality theory combines learning principles, modeling, cognition, and the effects of social relationships.

Locus of control refers to people's very general, cross-situational beliefs about what determines whether or not they get reinforced in life. People can be classified along a continuum from very internal to very external. People with a strong internal locus of control believe that the responsibility for whether or not they get reinforced ultimately lies with themselves. Internals believe that success or failure is due to their own efforts. In contrast, externals believe that the reinforcers in life are controlled by luck, chance, or powerful others. Therefore, they see little impact of their own efforts on the amount of reinforcement they receive.

External locus of control: perception that chance or external forces beyond personal control determine one's fate **Internal locus of control:** perception that you control your own fate.

Rotter has written extensively on problems with people's interpretations of the locus of control concept. First, he has warned people that locus of control is not a typology. It is not an either/or proposition. Second, because locus of control is a generalized expectancy it will predict people's behaviour across situations. However, there may be some specific situations where people, for example, who are generally external behave like internals. That is because their learning history has shown them that they have control over the reinforcement they receive in certain situations, although overall they perceive little control over what happens to them. Again, one can see the importance of conceiving of personality as the **interaction** of the person and the environment.

Learned Helplessness: a sense of hopelessness in which a person thinks that he/she is unable to prevent aversive events.

Rotter claimed that behaviour is determined by two major types of "expectancy": the expected outcome of a behaviour and the value a person places on that outcome.

Evaluation of social-cognitive theories

- Social-cognitive theories tend to be overly-mechanical.
- Overemphasizes environmental influences; gives little or no consideration to the possibility of innate personality differences or the effects of genetics.
- Does not recognize internal human qualities such as hope, aspiration, love, self-sacrifice.

Humanistic Theories

Its roots are based in existential psychology. Two American psychologists, Abraham Maslow and Carl Rogers paved the way for this new approach to understanding personality. When conflict between war and peace arose in the early to mid 1960s, so to did the need to understand human nature. Humanistic theory gave us an understandable way to look at man's need for war for the sake of peace. The basic ideas behind humanistic psychology are simple, some may say overly simple. Humanists hold the following beliefs:

1. The present is the most important aspect of the person and therefore humanists focus on the here and now rather than looking at the past or trying to predict the future.
2. Humanistic theory is reality based and to be psychologically healthy people must take responsibility for themselves, whether the person's actions are positive or negative.
   (a) The individual, merely by being human, posses an inherent worth. Actions may not be positive but this does not negate the value of the person.
   (b) The goal of life should always be to achieve personal growth and understanding. Only through self-improvement and self-knowledge can one truly be happy.

Abraham Maslow emphasized the basic goodness of human nature and a natural tendency toward self-actualization.

Abraham Maslow is considered father of the humanistic movement. He observed the lives of (purportedly) healthy and creative people to develop his theory. **Hierarchy of needs:** the motivational component of Maslow's theory, in which our innate needs, which motivate our actions, are hierarchically arranged. **Self-actualization:** the fullest realization of a person's potential. He viewed human needs or motives as forming a hierarchy. *Physiological needs:* At the bottom are the basic, primitive needs for air, food, water—those things we have to survive. *Safety and physical security needs:* shelter from weather, e.g., protection against tigers etc. *Love and belongingness needs:* Companionship, acceptance from others, affection. *Esteem needs:* needs for a sense of mastery and power. Need for appreciation from others. *Self-actualization:* The tendency to become whatever you are capable of becoming.The highest of human motives. In trying to describe the process of self-actualization.

Maslow: Self-actualizing people

Characteristics of self-actualized people according to Maslow (1968):

- efficient and accurate in perceiving reality
- are accepting of themselves, of other people and of nature
- are spontaneous in thought and emotion, rather than artificial

- are independent and autonomous
- identify with all of humanity and are democratic and respectful of others
- form very deep ties but only with a few people
- appreciate for its own sake the process of doing things
- have a childlike and fresh creativity and inventiveness
- maintain an inner detachment from the culture in which they live
- may appear temperamental or ruthless as they are strong and independent people guided by their own inner visions.

Maslow: Problems of measuring self-actualisation

It is hard for theorists to agree precisely WHAT self-actualization is and HOW to measure it. In other words it is not been tightly defined and operationalised. The concept of self-actualization provides some very interesting insights but it is hard to actually verify self-actualization scientifically. One scale, the Personal Orientation Inventory (POI) by Shostrom (1974), is a self-report measure of self-actualization. research using this measure finds the scale has various validity and reliability weaknesses but does at least capture some aspects of a healthy personality (e.g. Burwick & Knapp, 1991).

Rogers believed that the organism has one basic tendency and striving—to actualize, maintain, and enhance the experiencing organism. Rogers believed that all people have a tendency toward growth—Actualization. Rogers maintains that the human "organism" has an underlying "actualizing tendency", which aims to develop all capacities in ways that maintain or enhance the organism and move it toward autonomy. This tendency is directional, constructive and present in all living things. The actualizing tendency can be suppressed but can never be destroyed without the destruction of the organism (Rogers, 1977). The concept of the actualizing tendency is the only motive force in the theory. It encompasses all motivations; tension, need, or drive reductions; and creative as well as pleasure-seeking tendencies. There is a need to maintain and enhance life. The goal of existence is to satisfy this need. This desire to preserve and enhance oneself is on one level:

- Physical—staying alive by eating, keeping warm, avoiding physical danger etc. On a higher level:
- Psychological—self-actualization is about testing and fulfilling our capabilities: seek out new experiences, master new skills, quit boring jobs and find more exciting ones etc.

To the course of pursuing self-actualization, people engage in what Rogers called the organismic valuing process. Experiences perceived as not enhancing are valued as bad and are avoided. The best known and probably the most popular humanistic therapy is Rogers client-centred therapy. The therapist tries to see the world through the client's eyes so that the client will come to see his or her view of reality as having value.

The human organism's "phenomenal field" includes all experiences available at a given moment, both conscious and unconscious. As development occurs, a portion of this field becomes differentiated and this becomes the person's "self" (Hall and Lindzey, 1985; Rogers, 1959). The "self" is a central construct in this theory. It develops through interactions with others and involves awareness of being and functioning.

Evaluation of Humanistic Theories

- Many of the Humanists' claims are untestable.
- Humanists may have an overly-positive, rosy view of human kind. They do not look at the "dark side."
- For the Humanists, the cause of all our problems lies not in ourselves, but in others.

ALTERATION IN PERSONALITY

Most of people have abnormal behaviour classified as personality disorder. Let's take a look at several personality disorders.

Histrionic Personality Disorder

It is found more often in women than men. This disorder exhibits immature, self-centered, seductive, attentive-getting behaviour. People with this disorders are likely to be manipulative, a knack for making others feel guilty for one's awful sufferings. Such persons are flamboyant. They exaggerate how "truly wonderful" good things are and how "deeply tragic" bad things are. They also deny the sexual connotations of their seductive behaviour. The histrionic pattern may also include imagined ailments or illnesses that actually have psychological origins. Such ailments were treated by Freud. They may dress provocatively or exaggerate illnesses in order to gain attention. They also tend to exaggerate friendships and relationships, believing that everyone loves them.

Antisocial Personality Disorder

This disorder exhibits cheating behaviour needlessly, lying without reason, are suspicious of others and respond passively to others. They are selfish, irresponsible, impulsive, guiltless, and do not learn from puilishment. They are not fearful or addicts but their behaviour seems to be odd or abnormal which is a source of distress for themselves and others. This is also known as 'sociopathy' and 'psychopathy'. These symptoms are described by J.C. Prichard in 1837. He called it moral insanity because the intellect of such persons was normal but the moral values were deprived. He felt that such persons lack self discipline. The American psychological Association coined the term anti-social personality in late 1960's.

Characteristics of anti-social persons

1. Lack of moral values, anxiety and guilt
2. Irresponsible and impulsive behaviour
3. Superficial charm and efficient rationalist
4. Rejection of authority and inability to profit from experience
5. Unresponsive in general interpersonal relationships

Paranoid Personality Disorder

Paranoid personality disorder is characterized by a distrust of others and a constant suspicion that people around you have sinister motives. They search for hidden meanings in everything and read hostile intentions into the actions of others. They are quick to challenge the loyalties of friends and loved ones and often appear cold and distant to others. They usually shift blame to others and tend to carry long grudges. It is important to note that paranoid personalities are not psychotic, they are in sync with the reality most of the time although they may experience transient psychotic symptoms.

Borderline Personality Disorder

Borderline personalities are characterized by mood instability and poor self-image. People with this disorder are prone to constant mood swings arid bouts of anger. They will take their anger out on themselves, causing themselves injury. Suicidal threats and actions are not uncommon. They are often quick to anger when their expectations are not met. They have highly unstable sense of self and also have highly unstable interpersonal relationships. They tend to have low tolerance for frustration as well as chronic feelings of emptiness.

Narcissistic Personality Disorder

Narcissistic personalities are characterized by self-centeredness. They exaggerate their achievements, expecting others to recognize them as being superior. They have increased sense of self-importance, a preoccupation with being admired by others and lack of empathy for the feelings of others. They tend to be choosy about picking friends, since they believe that not just anyone is worthy of being their friend. They are generally uninterested in the feelings of others and may take advantage of them. This disorder is found more in men than women.

Schizoid Personality Disorder

People with schizoid personality disorder avoid relationships and do not show much emotion. They genuinely prefer to be alone and do not secretly wish for popularity. They tend to seek jobs that require little social contact. Their social skills are often weak and they do not show a need for attention or acceptance. They are perceived as humorless and distant and often are termed "loners." They may even appear indifferent to praise or criticism from others. In general, they do not experience any strong positive or negative emotions towards anyone.

They are aloof and cold.

Schizotypal Personality Disorder

Schizotypal personality is characterized by a need for social isolation, odd behaviour and thinking, and often unconventional beliefs such as being convinced of having extra sensory abilities. Some people believe that schizotypal personality disorder is a mild form of schizophrenia. They not only have social and interpersonal deficits but also experience cognitive and perceptual distortions and eccentricities in their communication and behaivour.

Avoidant Personality Disorder

Avoidant personality disorder is characterized by a pervasive pattern of social inhibition, feelings of inadequacy, and extreme sensitivity to negative evaluation. Individuals with this disorder consider themselves to be socially inept or personally unappealing, and avoid social interaction for fear of being ridiculed or humiliated. Some studies show that this disorder is biologically based, often starts in infancy or childhood and reinforced by environmental factors. A dependent personality has great difficulty in separating in relationships while an avoidant personality has problems in initiating relationships.

Dependent Personality Disorder

Dependent personality is characterized by a pervasive psychological dependence on other people. They have difficulty in making everyday decisions without an excessive amount of advice and reassurance from others. They fear to get appropriately angry with other people as they feel they may loose them. They lack self-confidence and feel helpless even when they have achieved good work skills or competencies.

Obsessive Compulsive Personality Disorder

Obsessive compulsive personality is characterized by a general psychological inflexibility, rigid conformity to rules and procedures, perfectionism, and excessive orderliness. People with OCPD tend to stress perfectionism above all else, and feel anxious when they perceive that things aren't "right". They are preoccupied with maintaining psychological and interpersonal control through careful attention to rules and time-table.. They are quite inflexible about moral and ethical issues. Other people tend to view them rigid, stiff and cold.

PSYCHOLOGICAL ASSESSMENTS OF PERSONALITY

Projective Test

Assessing the Unconscious *Projective Tests* used to assess personality (e.g., Rorschach or TAT tests). It provides ambiguous stimuli and subject projects his or her motives into the ambiguous stimuli. For example:

Rorschach Inkblot Test

It is the most widely used projective test and a set of 10 inkblots designed by Hermann Rorschach.

Assessing the Unconscious—Rorschach used to identify people's inner feelings by analyzing their interpretations of the blots.

Free association

Patient reports anything that comes to his/her mind. The psychoanalyst listens for links and themes that might tie the patient's fragmentary thoughts or remarks together.

Dream analysis

Dreams have two types of content:

- **Manifest content**—actual events in dream.
- **Latent content**—hidden message in dream.

Freud thought that each dream represents a form of wish fulfillment. The wish may be disguised, but it is always there.

Transference

Feelings of love or other emotions (hatred) are expressed toward the therapist. These feelings are actually unconsciously felt toward others; the patient is projecting these feelings onto the therapist. This provides clues about the client's feelings about these other people.

Thematic Apperception Test (TAT)

People express their inner motives through the stories they make up about ambiguous

MMPI-Minnesota multiphasic personality inventory

This is a personality test used as a clinical tool based on nomothetic approach. It was constructed by Hathaway and Kinley in 1943 and published by Minnesota Press. In 1945, the Psychological corporation was licensed to publish it. The MMPI is based on trait and type approach to personality. Ten clinical scales yield trait inferences in themselves. These scales give descriptive terms for behavioural disposition which may be of several kinds. MMPI can yield 19 profile types, each profile type contains several traits. It is remarkably robust and applicable in a wide-range of cultures. The test is useful for assessing degree of depression or anxiety or suicidal risk or ego strength or potential for impulsive behaviour. It can be used to supplement the information obtained through interview. The test's greatest utility is as an aid to patient assessment and it is also a powerful aid available. In the hands of an expert it can provide considerable valid and clinically useful information about emotional status of a cooperative subject.

16PF—Sixteen personality factor questionnaire

This is an objectively scorable test devised by Cattell. This test gives a comprehensive coverage of personality. It measures sixteen functionally independent and psychologically meaningful dimensions isolated and replicated in more than thirty years of factor analytic research on normal and clinical groups. Each factor is listed with its alphabetic designation and brief descriptions of low and high scores. 16PF is based on trait approach to personality. It gives the most comprehensive coverage of personality. Translations of the test into twentyfour languages and adaptations for five other English speaking cultures exist to facilitate international comparisons.

REFLECT YOURSELF

1. Write short note on personality disorders.
2. Discuss psychosexual stages.
3. Write a short note on approaches to study personality.

9

INTELLIGENCE

TOPICS COVERED IN THIS CHAPTER
• Introduction • Theories of Intelligence • Types of Intelligence Test • Uses of Intelligence Test • Concept of IQ

INTRODUCTION

Psychologists and laymen alike agree that a person who can reorganize and apply what he has acquired for the purpose of dealing with varied and novel situations is more intelligent than one who is capable of little beyond repeating what he had previously acquired or than one whose behaviour follows stereotyped patterns without insight into the essential elements and relations of each new situation. Since intelligence is a multifaceted concept it has been defined in varying ways. These definitions can be broadly classified into three categories:

One group of definitions says that it is adjustment or adaptation of the individual to his total environment or to limited aspects to it. According to definitions of this type, intelligence' is general mental adaptability to new problems and new situations of life. Thus, a more intelligent person is one who can more easily and more extensively vary his behaviour as changing conditions demand.

Second type of definitions state intelligence is the ability to learn. According to this type of definition, a person's intelligence is a matter of the extent to which he is educable. Thus, a more intelligent person will be readily and extensively able to learn and the greater is his possible range of experience and activity.

The third type of definitions states that intelligence is the ability to carry on the abstract thinking. This means the effective use of concepts and symbols in dealing with the situations especially a problem to be solved through the use of verbal and numerical symbols.

The two most acceptable definitions of intelligence are:

- "Intelligence is the aggregate or global capacity of the individual to act purposefully, to think rationally and to deal effectively with his environment." by Wechsler.
- "Intelligence is the ability to undertake activities that are characterized by(l)difficulty, (2) complexity, (3) abstractness, (4) economy, (5) adaptiveness to a goal (6) social value and (7) emergence of originals and to maintain such activities under conditions that demand a concentration of energy and a resistance to emotional force," by stoddard.

THEORIES OF INTELLIGENCE

Several theories have been developed to identify the different types of mental ability and to clarify the relationships among different abilities. These are:

- **Two factor theory:** was given by Charles Spearman in 1904. According to this theory, intelligence is comprised of '*g*' factor or general ability factor and '*s*' factor or specific ability factor. Spearman said that general ability factor is possessed by all individuals (in varying degrees due to individual differences) and operates in all mental activity (in varying amounts as mental tasks differ). Another factor is (s) which is required in specific amounts depending upon the mental task. This factor is independent of one's level of general intelligence. For *e.g.*, scores on a verbal comprehension test are determined largely by one's level of general intelligence but are also affected by one's specific ability to perform verbal comprehension tasks, independent of one's general intelligence.
- **Multifactor theory:** was given by E.L. Thorndike. According to this theory, intelligence is said to be constituted of a multitude of separate factors or elements each one being a minute element of ability. Any mental act, according to theory; involves a number of these minute elements operating together. Thorndike designed a CAVD test. This test is composed of four parts: sentence completion (C), arithmetical reasoning (A), vocabulary (V) and following directions (D). This test does not claim that these four sets of items encompass, the entire range of abstract intelligence but because of significant correlations between all types of measures within the tested range, it is held that other aspects of abstract intelligence can be estimated with satisfactory accuracy from those portions that are actually measured by this test.
- **Group factor theory:** was given by L. Thurstone. According to this theory, intelligent activity is not an expression of innumerable highly specific factors as Thorndike claimed. Nor is it the expression primarily of a general factor that pervades all mental activity and is the essence of intelligence as Spearman held. Instead, Thurstone's group factor theory emphasized on that certain mental operations have in common a 'primary' factor that gives them psychological and functional unity and that differentiates them from other mental operations. These mental operations then constitute a group. A second group of mental operations has its own unifying primary factor. The number is yet undetermined. Thurstone developed PMA (primary mental abilities) test. It includes 6 primary factors-verbal comprehension, word fluency, perceptual speed, memory, numerical ability, spatial ability and reasoning.
- **Hierarchical theories:** Vernon's Hierarchical model: suggests a general factor '*g*' which pervades all tests of intelligence and can be broken down into two categories called major group factors. These two major group factors are: verbal, educational and spatial-motor.

- **Guilford structure of intellect model:** Guilford does not accept the existence of a general intellectual factor, either in the basic sense proposed by Spearman or in the sense of a higher order factor as proposed by Vernon. Guilford proposes that intelligence is organised according to 3 dimensions.
    1. Operations: what a person does
    2. Contents: the material on which operations are performed
    3. Products: the form in which information is stored and processed.

  There are 5 types of operations, 4 types of content and 6 types of products. He proposed that each combination of a specific operation, a specific type of content and a specific type of product defines a unique type of intelligence. There are 120 different types of intelligence which he designed it in a cube.
- **Fluid and crystallised intelligence:** Cattell has suggested 2 distinct aspects of general intelligence ... fluid and crystallized. Fluid intelligence-refers to active mental energy to perceive relationships in any material, new or old, it reaches its maximum level at about fourteen or fifteen years as the brain finishes its growth. Whereas, Crystallized intelligence refers to the collection of skilled judgements as person has acquired by applying his fluid intelligence to his school opportunities. It refers to one's store of factual knowledge.
- **Process oriented theories of intelligence:** An alternate approach that uses different vocabulary, for e.g., instead of intelligence, theorists use the term 'cognition'. These are: Piaget's theory: intelligence is an adaptive process that involves an interplay of biological maturation and interaction with the environment. Bruner's theory: intellectual development partly as a growing reliance on internal representation. Young children know things by perceiving them and older children know things internally and symbollically *i.e.,* how they are able to devise internal symbols or representations of objects and actions and to hold these mental images in mind. He studied how environment plays an important role in developing intellectual skills. Information processing theories given by Sternberg proposed that intelligence can be broken down into basic skills that people employ to take in information, process it, and then use it to reason and solve problem.

Since intelligence is a complex concept, it comprises of varieties of components of intelligence. There have been varieties of tests which are designed to measure/assess intelligence. These are:

TYPES OF INTELLIGENCE TESTS

Mode of administration includes individual and group tests.

1. Individual tests: Stanford Binet Intelligence Scale, Wechsler Adult Intelligence Scale
2. Group tests: Cattell's Culture Fair Test, Scale 2, Raven's Progressive Matrices Scale 2

Type of content includes performance and paper and pencil tests

1. Performance tests: Wechsler Performance Scale
   Performance test of Intelligence by Bhatia
2. Paper and pencil tests: Cattel's Culture Fair Test

USES AND APPLICATIONS OF INTELLIGENCE TESTS

1. Intelligence tests may be widely used for the purpose of vocational guidance and counselling.
2. Identification of intellectual abilities for education purpose that may serve as devises to categorize individual and distinguish them between the intellectually superior, average or mentally retarded or inferior students, students requiring special attention and training.
3. The level of intelligence is often used as a criterion for selecting in specific jobs, occupation or field.
4. Intelligence tests help in the diagnosis of intellectual disturbance and maladjustments resulting from retardation.
5. Other than these intelligence tests, find extensive use in the armed services, industry, educational and research institution.

CONCEPT OF IQ

IQ means intelligence quotient, obtained by MA/CA *100. MA refers to mental age and CA refers to chronological age. Intellectual disorder can be classified as below:

50–69 mild mental retardation

35–49 moderate mental retardation

20–34 severe mental retardation

Under 20 profound mental retardation

Mild mental retardation refers to the people who acquire language with some delay but most achieve the ability to use speech for everyday purposes, to hold conversations and to engage in a clinical interview. Such people can engage in self care. Main difficulties are seen in academic school work, and many have particular problems in reading and writing. They can be helped though education.

Moderate mental retardation refers to the people whose skills in self care and motor skills is also retarded and some need supervision throughout life. Progress in academic work is limited. Their development in comprehension and use of language is also limited.

Severe mental retardation refers to marked degree of motor impairment or other associated deficits, indicating the presence of clinically significant damage to or maldevelopment of the central nervous system. This category is somewhat similar to the moderate mental retardation category.

Profound mental retardation refers to those affected individuals who are severely limited in their ability to understand or comply with requests or instructions. Such individuals are immobile and capable at most of only very rudimentary forms of nonverbal communication. They cannot engage in self-care and require constant help.

REFLECT YOURSELF

1. Discuss the concept of IQ.
2. Write a short note on nature of intelligence.
3. Discuss different types of intelligence tests.

10

APTITUDE

TOPICS COVERED IN THIS CHAPTER
• Concept of Aptitude • Types

CONCEPT OF APTITUDE

By aptitude we mean, one's potentialities at present as revealed by his performance for the future. DAT manual carries the definition of aptitude which Bingham prepared for Warren's Dictionary of Psychology.

"Aptitude is a condition or set of characteristics regarded as symptomatic of an individual's ability to acquire with training some (usually specified) knowledge, skill or set of responses, such as the ability to speak a language, to produce music ...."

According to Freeman, "aptitude is a combination of characteristics indicative of an individual's capacity to acquire (with training), some specific knowledge, skill or set of organized responses, such as the ability to speak a language, to become a musician or to do a mechanical work."

Aptitude is the result of interaction of heredity and environment. An individual is born with certain potentialities and begins to learn immediately. Aptitude is stable in life. It manifests in efficiency.

TYPES

- It is important to note that aptitude tests are different from intelligence tests or tests of skill and proficiency. Intelligence is a general mental ability. According to Thorndike, Guilford, Thurstone, intelligence is not a unitary trait. It is composed of different abilities. A single score on such tests will not uncover individual's potentialities in different abilities. Skill refers to the ability to perform a given test with ease and precision. Proficiency has much the same meaning except that it is more comprehensive for it to include not only skills in certain types of activities as shown by the extent of one's competence in language, book keeping, history, economics and maths. Whereas, aptitude tests are given to the individual in order to obtain the measure of his promise or essential teachability in a given area." Freeman.

- They do not measure ability that depends upon formal learning or training.
- DAT is one of them.
- It consists of eight independent tests. These are:
- **Verbal reasoning test:** it is a measure of ability to understand concepts framed in words. It evaluates student's ability to abstract or generalize and to think constructively.
- **Numerical ability test:** tests the understanding of numerical relationships and facility of handling numerical concepts.lt is a measure of the student's ability to reason with numbers, to manipulate numerical relationships and to deal intelligently with quantitative materials.
- **Abstract reasoning test:** assesses the ability to perceive relationships in abstract figure patterns-generalizations and education of principles from non-language designs.
- **Clerical speed and accuracy test:** it is designed to measure student's speed and accuracy with simple number and letter combinations. In this test , objective is to measure speed of perception, momentary retention and speed of response.
- **Mechanical reasoning test:** In this test, each item consists of pictorially presented mechanical situation together with a simply worded question.
- **Space relations test:** Measures the ability to deal with concrete materials through visualization. Space relations ability involve ability to manipulate things mentally, to create a structure in one's mind from a plan is what the test is designed to evaluate.
- **Test of spelling and language usage:** every item in the test contributes to its appropriate share which enhances the reliability of the test. The section on sentences of this test is intended to measure the ability to distinguish between good/bad grammar, punctuation and word usage.

REFLECT YOURSELF

1. Discuss what do you mean by aptitude? Or write a short note on different types of aptitude.

11

MOTIVATION

TOPICS COVERED IN THIS CHAPTER
• Introduction • Theories of Motivation • Types of Motivation

INTRODUCTION

Sania dreams of making big in hospitality industry for which she has started taking care of her diet and polishing her soft skills like communication. On Sundays along with gyming she attends English classes as well. Now what do you infer from such a behaviour. As a psychologist one would say that it is her motivation which keeps her focused and occupied in creating a niche in her chosen field of interest. What is motivation? Let us see how this concept is conceptualized by various researchers.

Motivation is a term used to refer to the driving and pulling forces which result in persistent behaviour directed towards particular goals. A general term for process of starting, directing and maintaining physical, and psychological activities. It is closely linked to all aspects of behaviour performance, learning, problem solving, etc. It is evidenced in persistence of organized patterns of activity toward desired relevant goals.

Motivational concepts are useful in accounting for:

- Variability in behaviour between people and within the person from time to time.
- Assigning responsibility for actions
- In relating behaviour with biological states
- In predicting behaviour
- In explaining behaviour that cannot be readily interpreted in terms of the current conditions in a situation.

THEORIES OF MOTIVATION

Instinct Theory

Starting with the Darwin's ideas, many psychologists believed that human beings have instinct. Mc. Dougall gave a list of instincts underlying human behaviour. Freud proposed two basic instincts: life instinct and death instinct.

Criticisms

- Behaviourists pointed out that many behaviours were learnt.
- Anthropologists found differences in behaviour in different cultures.

Drive Theory

It is a theory of motivation which suggests that behaviour is pushed from within by drives stemming from basic physiological needs. According to this view, states of deprivation arising our body create unpleasant states of arousal or drives the subjective feelings associated with needs (e.g., hunger, fatigue, etc) in order to eliminate such feelings and restore a balanced physiological state known as homeostasis we engage in certain activities. Furthermore, behaviours which reduce drives are strengthened and tend to be repeated.

In this view motivation is said to consist of :

- driving state
- the goal directed behaviour initiated by the drive state
- the attainment of an appropriate goal
- the reduction of the driving state
- after a time the driving state builds up again is called motivational cycle.

A original drive theory focussed on biological needs. Other theorists also included drives for stimulation such as status, wealth, power, etc., or which are learnt. Freud considered driving state to be inborn, instinctual and even based his ideas of personality on inborn sexual and aggressive urges or drives.

Drawbacks

(a) Curiosity motive not explained.

(b) It is seen that people often behave in ways that increase drives rather than reduce them. Eg. Skipping a snack to increase enjoyment of a meal.

(c) All behaviours are not driven by internal states. External objects or incentives also motivate behaviour.

Drive theories apply best to some of the biological motives.

Arousal Theory

According to this theory people seek an optimal level of arousal which varies from person to person as well as for different tasks. The theory focuses on arousal our general level of activation which varies from time to time and is reflected in such physiological measures as heart rate, bp, brain activity, muscle tension, etc., according to this theory, we seek not minimal levels but optimal level of arousal a level that is suitable for our personal characteristics as well as the kind of task we are currently doing.

Support for the theory

Weiner (1989) finds close link between performance and arousal. Highest performance at moderate levels of arousal. However, it is difficult to determine in advance what level of arousal will be optimal for a given task. Zuckerman (1984) found that large individual differences in preferred level of arousal. People report both feeling well and performing well under optimal arousal condition. The theory is able to explain why people often seek to higher arousal.

Expectancy Theory

A cognitive approach. This theory suggests that behaviour is pulled by expectations of desired outcomes. Many behaviours are resorted to not because they reduce biological drives but because we expect that the behaviour will lead to achieving important goals in the future. Such outcomes are also termed as incentives. Common incentives are money, status, power, admiration.

- Application of expectancy theory primarily in work motivation in industrial/organizational psychology.
- Incentives have an activating/energizing effect on behaviour that occur before a goal is reached in a way they are like reinforcements which are in anticipation of goal/rewards.
- Thus, behaviour is motivated not by objective reality but our interpretation of reality.
- Our present behaviour is controlled by
  —what we think caused by past successes,
  —what we believe it is possible for us to do,
  —what we anticipate will be outcome of an action.

TYPES OF MOTIVATION

Aggressive Motivation

It is the desire to harm or injure others in some manner. Is aggression an innate tendency or externally elicited behaviour? Freud's view-we share an aggressive instinct with lower animals. Freud also believed that desire to hurt or be hurt by one's sexual partner are normal in humans. Studies do support the view that portions of human brain regulate expressions of aggression and that levels of hormones (testesterone) are related to aggression. Aggression is perceived as abstract, or unjustified (Zillman and Cantor, 1976). Aggression may be due to unpleasant, aversive environmental conditions such as high temperature, intense noise and crowding. Berkowitz negative effect i.e., unpleasant feelings aroused by environmental or social situations can trigger emotions, thoughts, and memories of aggression.

Social learning theory

Bandura (1987): role of initiation of others behaviour e.g., aggressive models. Modeling is an important cause of aggressive behaviour because:

(a) It directs observers attention to all possible behaviour
(b) Shows observer that certain behaviours are restraints and all right. Lowers inhibition to aggression.
(c) Enhances emotional arousal which might facilitate aggression under certain conditions.
(d) Shows observer some specific behaviour that might be copied.

(e) Distorting views about conflict resolution.
- Classical conditioning and instrumental conditions can be important sources of human aggression. e.g., hostility and aggression towards father may even generalize to other authority figures and if aggression pays off it may become habitual in certain situations.
- Aggressive expressions and catharsis —2 views:
  (a) Expression of aggression should be cathartic i.e., reduce intensity of aggression.
  (b) Expression of aggression leads to increased aggressive behaviour if reinforced.

Achievement Motivation

Murray (1938) postulated 'need to achieve' achievement motivation refers to desire to accomplish difficult task and to meet standard of excellence. According to Smith 1969; Spence and Helmreich 1983: achievement is task oriented behaviour that allows the individual performance to be evaluated according to some internally or externally imposed criterion that involves the individual in competing with others or that otherwise involves some standards of excellence.

Sources of ach motivation

(a) Imitation of models, observational learning (Bandura and Walkers 1963)

(b) Emphasis of parents as excellence and expectations of parents regarding becoming independent.

(c) Encouraging children to take credit for their success *i.e.,* to attribute the child's success to the child's own efforts.

People with high achievement motivation work longer and harder on difficult tasks whereas low achievement motivation people will give up on a difficult task.

High achievers in organization have higher level of motivation.

Power Motivation

It is the motivation to intent to have high status and exert influence over others. Winter (1973) has defined social power as the ability or capacity of a person to extended effects on the behaviour or emotions of another person. Machiavellianism: is a term used to describe people who express their power motivation by manipulating and exploiting others in a deceptive and unscrupulous manner.

Biological Motives

The arousal of biological motives is disruption of homoestasis. This initiates both automatic processes and motivated behaviour to restore equilibrium. Hormones or chemical messengers circulating in the blood also arouse biological motive states.

Factors which regulate eating and hunger :

(a) Detector cells in the hypothalamus, liver , blood, etc.

(b) Feedback produced by chewing and swallowing.

(c) Smell, taste and insight of food.

(d) Learning and experience.

(e) Cognitive factors: presence of others, emotional factor and personality.

REFLECT YOURSELF

1. What are the different types of motivation?
2. Write a short note on theories of motivation.

12

EMOTION

TOPICS COVERED IN THIS CHAPTER
• Introduction • Components of Emotion • Emotional Adjustment • What is Good Emotional Health? • How can my Emotions Affect my Health? • Why does my Doctor Need to Know About my Emotions? • How can I Improve my Emotional Health? • How the Concept of Emotion is Conceptualized?

INTRODUCTION

Today my father gave me a football to play. I am feeling very happy and I started playing hard with it. After few moments it went into the canal. Now I am very sad. I wonder what does it child means by being happy and sad. What is emotion? Is it a feeling? Then what is a feeling? These terms are difficult to define and even more difficult to understand completely. People have been attempting to understand this phenomenon for thousands of years, and will most likely debate for a thousand more. The mainstream definition of emotion refers to a feeling state involving thoughts, physiological changes, and an outward expression or behaviour. But what comes first? The thought? The physiological arousal? The behaviour? Or does emotion exist in a vacuum, whether or not these other components are present? There are five theories which attempt to understand why we experience emotion.

Definition of emotion: Emotion is the language of a person's internal state of being, normally based in or tied to their internal (physical) and external (social) sensory feeling. Love, hate, courage, fear, joy, and sadness can all be described in both psychological and physiological terms: Emotion is the realm where thought and physiology are inextricably entwined, and where the 'self is inseparable from our individual perceptions of value and judgement toward ourselves and toward others in our emotional space.

COMPONENTS OF EMOTION

Three components of emotion:

1. Physiological: arousal comes from the brain (particularly the limbic system) and autonomic nervous system (ANS). It refers to disruption of homeostatic baselines. For e.g., when you experience emotion of fear, your pulse rate and heart begins to rise.
2. Cognitive: thoughts, values and expectations. The cognitive aspect of emotion involves thoughts a particular person has when they are experiencing a particular emotion. For example: if you are feeling happy you may say to yourself, what a wonderful day today is.
3. Behavioural: expressions, gestures and body positions. The behavioural aspect of emotion involves people to take actions when they experience emotion. For example; if you are feeling happy you might hug the person next to you. Or if you are afraid of something you might run away from it.

Experiencing an emotion has an effect on you: the way you think, functioning of your body and the way you behave.

EMOTIONAL ADJUSTMENT

- **Emotional adjustment** (also referred to as **personal adjustment or psychological adjustment)** is the maintenance of emotional equilibrium in the face of internal and external stressors. This is facilitated by cognitive processes of acceptance and adaptation. An example would be maintaining emotional control and coping behaviour in the face of an identity crisis. This capacity is an important aspect of mental health and where it is compromised, or not developed, psychopathology and mental disorder can result.

WHAT IS GOOD EMOTIONAL HEALTH?

People who have good emotional health are aware of their thoughts, feelings and behaviours. They have learned healthy ways to cope with the stress and problems that are a normal part of life. They feel good about themselves and have healthy relationships.

However, many things that happen in your life can disrupt your emotional health and lead to strong feelings of sadness, stress or anxiety. These things include:

- Being laid off from your job
- Having a child leave or return home
- Dealing with the death of a loved one
- Getting divorced or married
- Suffering an illness or an injury
- Getting a job promotion
- Experiencing money problems

- Moving to a new home
- Having a baby

"Good" changes can be just as stressful as "bad" changes

HOW CAN MY EMOTIONS AFFECT MY HEALTH?

Your body responds to the way you think, feel and act. This is often called the "mind/body connection." When you are stressed, anxious or upset, your body tries to tell you that something isn't right. For example, high blood pressure or a stomach ulcer might develop after a particularly stressful event, such as the death of a loved one. The following can be physical signs that your emotional health is out of balance:

- Back pain
- Change in appetite
- Chest pain
- Constipation or diarrhoea
- Drymouth
- Extreme tiredness
- General aches and pains
- Headaches
- High blood pressure
- Insomnia (trouble sleeping)
- Lightheadedness
- Palpitations (the feeling that your heart is racing)
- Sexual problems
- Shortness of breath
- Stiffneck
- Sweating
- Upset stomach
- Weight gain or loss

Poor emotional health can weaken your body's immune system, making you more likely to get colds and other infections during emotionally difficult times. Also, when you are feeling stressed, anxious or upset, you may not take care of your health as well as you should. You may not feel like exercising, eating nutritious foods or taking medicine that your doctor prescribes. Abuse of alcohol, tobacco or other drugs may also be a sign of poor emotional health.

WHY DOES MY DOCTOR NEED TO KNOW ABOUT MY EMOTIONS?

You may not be used to talking to your doctor about your feelings or problems in your personal life. But remember, he or she can't always tell that you're feeling stressed, anxious or upset just by looking at you. It's important to be honest with your doctor if you are having these feelings.

First, he or she will need to make sure that other health problems aren't causing your physical symptoms. If your symptoms aren't caused by other health problems, you and your doctor can address the emotional causes of your symptoms. Your doctor may suggest ways to treat your physical symptoms while you work together to improve your emotional health.

If your negative feelings don't go away and are so strong that they keep you from enjoying life, it's especially important for you to talk to your doctor. You may have what doctors call "major depression." Depression is a medical illness that can be treated with individualized counseling, medicine or with both.

HOW CAN I IMPROVE MY EMOTIONAL HEALTH?

First, try to recognize your emotions and understand why you are having them. Sorting out the causes of sadness, stress and anxiety in your life can help you manage your emotional health. The following are some other helpful tips.

Express your Feelings in Appropriate Ways

If feelings of stress, sadness or anxiety are causing physical problems, keeping these feelings inside can make you feel worse. It's OK to let your loved ones know when something is bothering you. However, keep in mind that your family and friends may not be able to help you deal with your feelings appropriately. At these times, ask someone outside the situation—such as your family doctor, a counselor or a religious advisor—for advice and support to help you improve your emotional health.

Live a Balanced Life

Try not to obsess about the problems at work, school or home that lead to negative feelings. This doesn't mean you have to pretend to be happy when you feel stressed, anxious or upset. It's important to deal with these negative feelings, but try to focus on the positive things in your life too. You may want to use a journal to keep track of things that make you feel happy or peaceful. Some research has shown that having a positive outlook can improve your quality of life and give your health a boost. You may also need to find ways to let go of some things in your life that make you feel stressed and overwhelmed. Make time for things you enjoy.

Develop Resilience

People with resilience are able to cope with stress in a healthy way. Resilience can be learned and strengthened with different strategies. These include having social support, keeping a positive view of yourself, accepting change and keeping things in perspective.

Calm your Mind and Body

Relaxation methods, such as meditation, are useful ways to bring your emotions into balance. Meditation is a form of guided thought. It can take many forms. For example, you may do it by exercising, stretching or breathing deeply. Ask your family doctor for advice about relaxation methods.

Take Care of Yourself

To have good emotional health, it's important to take care of your body by having a regular routine for eating healthy meals, getting enough sleep and exercising to relieve pent-up tension. Avoid overeating and don't abuse drugs or alcohol. Using drugs or alcohol just causes other problems, such as family and health problems.

HOW THE CONCEPT OF EMOTION IS CONCEPTUALIZED?

James Lange Theory

Felt emotion is the perception of bodily changes. William james and carl lange proposed the following sequence of events in emotional state. According to them, that subjective emotional experiences are actually the result of changes within our bodies. In other words, you feel frightened when making your speech because you notice that your heart is racing, etc. james said that "we feel sorry because we cry, angry because we strike.

Canon Bard Theory

Suggested that there are specific brain centers in the thalamic, hypothalamic regions which are responsible for emotional experiences. For example: when the student finds principal approaching the nerve impulses pass through the thalamus. From there some impulses are sent to the cortex where the stimulus is perceived and emotion is experienced, while other impulses travel to the muscles and viscera where the physiological changes occur. In contrast, to James Lange theory, emotion experience takes place because stimulus is perceived by the cortex. But according to James Lange theory emotional experience take place when the person perceives physiological changes that occur within the body. Secondly, Canon-bard suggested that both the experience of emotion and physiological changes occur at the same time, as a result of nervous activity in thalamus and hypothalamus.

Schachter Singer Theory

Emotions are caused by two components. These are physiological arousal which tends to be vague and diffused. Secondly, cognitive process by which individual label their physiological arousal through situational cues. S-S theory, emphasized the interaction between a person's thoughts and his/her physiological arousal. Thus, this theory showed a relation between emotion and cognition.

Theory of Relationships Among Emotion

Robert Plutchik, proposed a descriptive theory *i.e.*, concerned with what are called primary, basic emotions and the ways they can be mixed together. Plutchik, assumes that they are different in three ways:

(a) Intensity
(b) Similarity to one another
(c) Oppositeness or polarity

Using these three ways to distinguish between emotions he designed a spatial model. The strongest varieties of emotion are at the top of the segment with progressively weaker varities toward the bottom. Grief is strongest then sadness, polarity is shown by the arrangement of segments. Grief is opposite to ectasy. Similar emotions are placed near to each other.

Opponent Process Theory

Proposed by Solomon (1982). The theory has two central assumptions.

(a) Emotional reactions to a stimulus are followed automatically by an opposite reaction. (b) Repeated exposure to a stimulus causes the initial reaction to weaken and the opponent process to strengthen. For example, an individual who experience anxiety before making a public speech may when it is finished, experience strong feelings of relief. With repeated experience in public speaking, the anxiety may decrease while the feelings of relief and accomplishment will intensify.

Discrepancy Evaluation Theory

Proposed by Mandler. According to this theory, that arousal is produced by discrepancies between expected and actual events and that greater such arousal the more intense the emotion experienced. The level of arousal determines the intensity of the emotional experience; while cognitive evaluation determines its quality or specific identity, i.e., negative or positive emotion. For example; if you get a higher or lower grade on an exam than what you expected. The level of arousal in both cases will be high due to the impact of discrepancies. If the grade was better than what you had expected you label your arousal positively and feel proud and elated.

REFLECT YOURSELF

1. How the concept of emotion is conceptualized?
2. Write a short note on emotional adjustment.
3. What are the components of emotion?

13

STRESS

TOPICS COVERED IN THIS CHAPTER
• Introduction • Types of Stress • Eustress • Distress • Coping Strategies

INTRODUCTION

What is Stress?

Stress is your mind and body's response or reaction to a real or imagined threat, event or change. The threat, event or change are commonly called stressors. Stressors can be internal (thoughts, beliefs, attitudes or external (loss, tragedy, change).

According to Lazarus & Folkman, (1984): "stress is an internal state which can be caused by physical demands on the body (disease conditions, exercise, extremes of temperature and the like) or by environmental and social situations which are evaluated as potentially harmful, uncontrollable exceeding our resources for coping." A state of stress has two components: one is a stressor—the event that creates demands and stress response, a person's idiosyncratic reactions to the demands.

TYPES OF STRESS

(a) Frustration
(b) Conflicts and
(c) Pressures.

Frustration

occurs when one's strivings are thwarted, either by obstacles that block progress toward a desired goal or by absence of an appropriate goal. It may arise from internal or outer sources. *External frustration*: caused by scarcity of resources, famines, droughts, death of a loved ones, stringent rules of the society, physical violence, punishments imposed on breaking the rules, lack of opportunity, etc. *Effect*: such stressors evoke feelings of inadequacy, isolation, insecurity. *Internal frustration*: caused by emotional conflict due to personal inadequacy, isolation, guilt, high ambition, etc. *Effect*: it can evoke inferiority complex and self devaluation.

Conflict

Arises when needs are opposed to each other. It can be classified as: Approach-avoidant: where there are strong tendencies both to approach and to avoid the same goal. Double-approach: involve competition between two or more desirable goals. Double avoidant: involve conflict where competition is between two or more undesirable goals.

Pressure

It is a third type of stress which is in the form of expectation and standards which usually one sets for him/herself or are set by others. It may be caused by one's level of aspiration, self-ideal and certain standards are expected in education, marriage, occupation, etc.

G.A.S.

Pioneering Researcher who studied and developed a theory about how stress produces illness was Hans Selye. He gave the concept of general adaptation syndrome popularly known as G.A.S. it has three stages.

Alarm

"Fight or Flight" reaction: body mobilizes resources to combat threat; activates the sympathetic nervous system. As you begin to experience a stressful event or perceive something to be stressful psychological changes occur in your body. This experience or perception disrupts your body's normal balance and your immediately body begins to respond to the stressor(s) as effectively as possible.

Examples:

- Cardiac–increased heart rate
- Respiratory–increased respiration
- Skin–decreased temperature
- Hormonal–increased stimulation of adrenal

Resistance

Enhanced ability to fight stressor via moderate physiological arousal; ability to withstand additional stressors (e.g., infection) is reduced. During this stage your body tries to cope or adapt to the stressors by beginning a process of repairing any damage the stressor has caused. Your friends, family or co-workers may notice changes in you before you do so it is important to examine their feedback to make sure you do not reach overload. Example: Behaviour indicators include: lack of enthusiasm for family, school, work or life in general, withdrawal, change in eating habits, insomnia, hypersomnia, anger, fatigue. Cognitive Indicators include: poor problem solving, confusion, nightmares, hyper-vigilance.

More examples include: tearfulness, fear, anxiety, panic, guilt, agitation, depression, overwhelmed.

Exhaustion

Depletion of resources brings on diseases and disorders (e.g., chronically high heart rate and blood pressure increase chances of heart attack and stroke). During this stage the stress not being managed effectively and the body and mind are not able to repair the damage produced by stress. **Examples:** Digestive disorders, withdrawal, headaches, tension and insomnia.

EUSTRESS

Eustress or positive stress occurs when your level of stress is high enough to move into action to get things accomplished. It is a good stress. The word, "Eu" Greek meaning good.

E.g: an attractive acquaintance asks for a date; a college Student makes it to the dean's list.

DISTRESS

Distress or negative stress occurs when your level of stress is either too high or too low and your body and/or mind begin to respond negatively to the stressors.

Burnout: the term given by Christina Maslach.

"burnout is a syndrome of emotional exhaustion, depersonalization and reduced personal accomplishment that can occur among individuals who do "people work" of some kind." it is a state of complete mental, physical and emotional exhaustion.

3 aspects of burnout: First, emotional exhaustion as emotional resources are depleted and workers feel that they no longer able to give of themselves at a psychological level.

Second, development of depersonalization i.e., -ve , cynical attitudes and feelings about one's clients involving dehumanized perception of others which can lead to staff members to view their clients as deserving of their troubles.

Third, reduced personal accomplishments. This refers to the tendency to evaluate oneself negatively, particularly with regard to one's work with clients.

Effects of burnout:

1. Workers may feel unhappy about themselves and dissatisfied with their accomplishments on the job.
2. Deterioration in the quality of care or service provided by the staff, leading to low morale absenteeism, job turnover.
3. Physical exhaustion, insomnia, increased use of alcohol and drugs.

COPING STRATEGIES

Problem-Focused Coping: a response aimed at reducing, modifying, or eliminating a source of stress. (e.g., if grades in a course are low, reduce work hours, change study strategy, etc.). Emotion-

Focused Coping: a response aimed at reducing the emotional impact of the stressor (e.g., denial, religious faith, wishful thinking, humor, alcohol/drugs, promiscuous sex). In the low grades example, you can reappraise the stressor and reduce the importance you attach to that course, that major, or academic work in general. Two major emotion-focused strategies are:

Meditation and biofeedback.

There are coping strategies at individual level. There are types of prevention:

- Primary prevention: where you do not allow a stressful situation to occur.
- Secondary prevention: a problem has occurred aud then you try to prevent yourself from effects that problem would cause.
- Tertiary prevention: a problem has occurred developed and now you take rehabilitating oneself after stress.

Goal of intervention are of 4 kinds.

Coping strategies at individual level: (A) biological level: one can eat balanced and nutritive diet. Biofeedback can be taught on how to monitor own body mechanisms. (B) physical: through exercise and yoga, reduces chances of heart disease and psychosomatic illness. (C) spiritual: healing through meditation. (D) social: through social networking. The more social network you have greater the likelihood of stress but not resulting into burnout. (E) emotional: ventilation through anger, cry, and laughter. (F) cognitive: rational/cognitive emotive therapies putting right your thoughts, remove self-defeating and bringing positive emotions.

It involves three stages:

1. Thought stopping
2. Combine negative thoughts with auto suggestion "I can"
3. Then replace it with something positive.

REFLECT YOURSELF

1. Write a short note on coping strategies.
2. How the concept of stress is conceptualized?

14

ATTITUDE

TOPICS COVERED IN THIS CHAPTER

- Introduction
- Measurement of Attitudes
- Attitude Theories
- Factors Affecting Attitude

INTRODUCTION

The defining nature of attitude is that they express an evaluation of some object, event or human or animal being. Attitudes can be formed about many things. The object of attitudes can be entities (a lecture, a restaurant, television programme), people (political leader, friends, or acquaintance or yourself) or abstract concepts (birth of a baby, rights, riots, etc). Indeed anything that arouses evaluative feelings qualifies as an object of attitudes. Attitudes differ from beliefs, or opinions. Beliefs are cognitions or thoughts, about the characteristics of objects. They link objects to attributes. Suppose your friend expresses favourable attitude towards girls. This attitude is associated with a number of specific beliefs about the girls—girls are innocent and highly intuitive, they are ranked highly on soft skills. Those who agree with this statements will increase in their likings for girls or who disagree will not like girls. Attitudes guide behaviour. This statement is highly contradictory. Suppose your friend like girls. You will interpret that he will do friendship with girls, idiolize some girl as his girlfriend, but contrary he never sits with girls, never talk and avoid the company of girls. In such a case, attitude is not guiding behaviour.

MEASUREMENT OF ATTITUDES

To measure attitudes, there are several methods. They vary from very simple to very complex. The simplest method is to place concepts, things or people into a "favourable" or unfavourable category.

The most common method of measuring attitudes is self-report method. In this method the people are asked to respond to questions by expressing their personal evaluations. One of the self report method is public opinion polling. Public opinion polls are used either to predict something or to provide information. They are used to predict outcomes of elections, the likelihood of buying a product, or the degree of public support for implementing new policies. They can also be used to provide information about the percentage of the population that supports the use of marijuana, the death penalty or a low cost housing project. The complexities of opinion polling can be reduced to four steps: (1) selecting a sample of respondents, (2) constructing the attitude items, (3) administering items to the sample and (4) tabulating the results. For self report methods, an attitude item consists of a question or statement about the object and a format for the response. The format can be either fixed, where the categories for the response are named, or open ended where respondents use their own words.

The galvanic skin response (GSR) was one of the first measures tried out. The GSR measures the electrical resistance of the skin. This resistance decreases when a person is emotionally aroused. Although some research has been successful in relating GSR changes to the extremity of attitudes, it has never been possible to distinguish extremely favourable from extremely unfavourable attitudes; both extremes produce changes in the GSR. Other indications of arousal, such as size of the pupils of the eye, might be used to gauge a person's attitude. Pupil size has not yet been established as a good way to measure attitudes.

ATTITUDE THEORIES

The theories most frequently used to describe attitude are:

(a) Learning theories
(b) Consistency theories or
(c) Cognitive response theories

It should be noted that these different approaches are not contradictory but simply focus on different factors which may affect the way attitudes develop and change.

Learning theories

Doob (1947) proposed that the principles of classical and instrumental conditioning could be used to explain the formation and change of attitudes in much the same way that they have been applied to overt behaviour. Objects, people or events associated with pleasant experience may take on favourable evaluations, while those associated with unpleasant experiences may be evaluated negatively. If you express an attitude to a friend who then provides positive reinforcement (by smiling) your attitude is likely to be strenghthened. On the other hand, if your friend provides punishment (by frowning, disagreeing or expressing disapproval), your attitude is likely to be weakened. Peer groups such as clubs, unions, fraternities and churches differentially reinforce the expression of certain attitudes relevant to the group.

Consistency theories

Balance theory involves the relations between a person and two attitude objects. The three elements are connected by either favourable (good, liking or positive) attitudes or unfavourable (bad, disliking, or negative) attitudes. In the first diagram Ram is favourable towards X and learns that Arav is also favourable. In the second diagram, both Ram and Arav are unfavourable toward candidate X.

The basic tenet of balance theory is that there is a tendency to maintain or restore balance in one's attitude structures. Unbalanced structures are somehow uncomfortable or unpleasant. The third diagram illustrates an unbalanced state. In this instance, balance theory predicts that Arav will try to restore balance by changing one or more of her attitudes. She may change her attitude toward candidate X, or she may decide she no longer likes Ram. She may also attempt to restore balance by trying to persuade Ram to change his attitude toward candidate X. many studies have demonstrated that people express a preference for balanced structures and "fill in" incomplete structures in such a way as to maintain balance.

Cognitive dissonance: in 1957, Leon Festinger published this theory. Like balance theory the focus of cognitive dissonance among the elements is in their cognitive or thought, structures. For Festinger, any two related cognitive elements will be dissonant, if they do not fit together because they violate general logic or the person's expectations. For example: "smoking is injurious to health". People holding this thought along with another thought that not everybody gets cancer or die because of smoking. It will cause dissonance in the mind of the individual. To balance the thoughts one will (1) change one of the cognitive elements and (2) to add a new cognitive element. If neither of these changes in cognitive element is made, the smoker may add a new element, such as switching to filter cigarettes.

Cognitive response theories

They focus on the fact that the recipient does more than react to the external information; the recipient also generates thoughts about the information. These thoughts can increase, neutralize, or even reverse the intended impact of the information. Greenwald suggested that when people receive a persuasive message, they relate the information in the message to their existing store of knowledge.

FACTORS AFFECTING ATTITUDE

1. *Source of the message*
   (a) Credibility of the source is related to expertness and trustworthiness. For example; a dentist recommends a particular brand of toothpaste would change the opinion of the patient as the person will rely on the doctor's advise.
   (b) Attractiveness of the source for example: a popular cine star is recommending a particular brand of shampoo, it has greater effect on the receiver than just the information about the good qualities of the same shampoo.
   (c) Style of presentation: include emphasis on certain words, changing the tone and pitch of the speech and gestures. Style of presentation depends upon the personality of the source. For example: the same source material taught different teachers result in different degrees of learning.
2. *Content of the message:* Messages contain words and other symbols that convey information. Persuaders of all sorts spend countless hours on their messages to make them successful in changing attitudes.
   (a) **Novelty:** the new information is generally more effective in attracting your attention than the routine one.

(b) **Emotional appeal:** messages that make the receiver feel good tend to be more effective because they evoke favourable response however, some message which arouse fears are also effective in order to prevent somebody indulging in something undesirable. However, research show that low threat messages are more persuasive than high threat messages because high threat leads to the blocking of the message. Also, much depends upon the credibility of the source.

(c) **Number of arguments:** depends upon the receiver. If the receiver is well informed then both the sides of the argument should be presented.

(d) **Suggestion:** if the message is designed in such a way that people will accept a belief, form an attitude or be incited to action by someone else say so (famous personality), without requiring facts.

3. *Characteristics of receiver*

(a) **Persuasibility:** C.L. Hovland and I.L.Janis contended that persuasibility is a personality trait. They found that people who are easily persuaded under one set of conditions, will often be easily persuaded under another.

(b) **Self-esteem:** W.J.Mc. Guire observed that people with low self-esteem do not value their own opinion and therefore, they easily give up under pressure.

REFLECT YOURSELF

1. Discuss factors affecting attitude.
2. Write short note on theories of attitude.

15

PSYCHOLOGY OF PEOPLE (AT DIFFERENT AGES—FROM INFACY TO OLD AGE)

TOPICS COVERED IN THIS CHAPTER

- Concept of Psychology
- Psychology at Different Ages

CONCEPT OF PSYCHOLOGY

Erikson believed that personality develops in a series of stages. Erikson's theory describes the impact of social experience across the whole lifespan. Our personality traits come in opposites. We think of ourselves as optimistic or pessimistic, independent or dependent, emotional or unemotional, adventurous or cautious, leader or follower, aggressive or passive. Many of these are inborn temperament traits, but other characteristics, such as feeling either competent or inferior, appear to be learned, based on the challenges and support we receive in growing up. The man who did a great deal to explore this concept is Erik Erikson. Although he was influenced by Freud, he believed that the ego exists from birth and that behaviour is not totally defensive. Erikson became aware of the massive influence of culture on behaviour and placed more emphasis on the external world, such as depression and wars. He felt the course of development is determined by the interaction of the body (genetic biological programming), mind (psychological), and cultural (ethos) influences. He organized life into eight stages that extend from birth to death (many developmental theories only cover childhood). Since adulthood covers a span of many years, Erikson divided the stages of adulthood into the experiences of young adults, middle aged adults and older adults. While the actual ages may vary considerably from one stage to another, the ages seem to be appropriate for the majority of people. Erikson's basic philosophy might be said to rest on two major themes: (1) the world gets bigger as we go along and (2) failure is cumulative. While the first point is fairly obvious, we might take exception to the last. However, there's always the chance that somewhere along the way the strength of the human spirit can be ignited and deficits overcome. As you read through the following eight stages with their sets of opposites, notice which strengths you identify with most and those you need to work on some more.

PSYCHOLOGY AT DIFFERENT AGES

Infancy: Birth to 18 Months

Ego development outcome: Trust vs. mistrust

Basic strength: Drive and hope

It is the most fundamental stage in life. Erikson also referred to infancy as the Oral Sensory Stage (as anyone might who watches a baby put everything in her mouth) where the major emphasis is on the mother's positive and loving care for the child, with a big emphasis on visual contact and touch. If we pass successfully through this period of life, we will learn to trust that life is basically okay and have basic confidence in the future. If we fail to experience trust and are constantly frustrated because our needs are not met, we may end up with a deep-seated feeling of worthlessness and a mistrust of the world in general. Incidentally, many studies of suicides and suicide attempts point to the importance of the early years in developing the basic belief that the world is trustworthy and that every individual has a right to be here. Not surprisingly, the most significant relationship is with the maternal parent, or whoever is our most significant and constant caregiver.

Early Childhood: 18 Months to 3 Years

Ego development outcome: Autonomy vs. shame

Basic strengths: Self-control, courage, and will

During this stage we learn to master skills for ourselves. Not only do we learn to walk, talk and feed ourselves, we are learning finer motor development as well as the much appreciated toilet training. Here we have the opportunity to build self-esteem and **autonomy** as we gain more control over our bodies and acquire new skills, learning right from wrong. And one of our skills during the "Terrible Two's" is our ability to use the powerful word "NO!" It may be pain for parents, but it develops important skills of the will. It is also during this. However, that we can be very vulnerable. If we're shamed in the process of toilet training However, Erikson's reasoning was quite different than that of Freud's. Erikson believes that learning to control one's body functions leads to a feeling of control and a sense of independence. Other important events include gaining more control over food choices, toy preferences, and clothing selection. Children who successfully complete this stage feel secure and confident, while those who do not are left with a sense of inadequacy and self-doubt or in learning other important skills, we may feel great **shame and doubt** of our capabilities and suffer low self esteem as a result. The most significant relationships are with parents.

Play Age: 3 to 5 Years

Ego development outcome: Initiative vs. guilt

Basic strength: Purpose

During this period we experience a desire to copy the adults around us and take **Initiative** in creating play situations. We make up stories with Barbie's and Ken's, toy phones and miniature cars, playing out roles in a trial universe, experimenting with the blueprint for what we believe it means to be an adult. We also begin to use that wonderful word for exploring the world-"WHY?" While Erikson was influenced by Freud, he down plays biological sexuality in favour of the psychosocial features of conflict between child and parents. Nevertheless, he said that at this stage we usually become involved in the classic "Oedipal struggle" and resolve this struggle through "social role identification." If we're frustrated over natural desires and goals, we may easily experience **guilt.** Children who are successful at this stage feel capable and able to lead others. Those who fail to acquire these skills are left with a sense of guilt, self-doubt and lack of initiative. The most significant relationship is with the basic family.

School Age: 6 to 12 Years

Ego development outcome: Industry vs. inferiority

Basic strengths: Method and competence

During this stage, often called the Latency, we are capable of learning, creating and accomplishing numerous new skills and knowledge, thus developing a sense of **industry.** This is also a very social stage of development and if we experience unresolved feelings of inadequacy and **inferiority** among our peers, we can have serious problems in terms of competence and self-esteem. As the world expands a bit, our most significant relationship is with the school and neighbourhood. Parents are no longer the complete authorities they once were, although they are still important.

Adolescence: 12 to 18 Years

Ego development outcome: Identity vs. role confusion

Basic strengths: Devotion and fidelity

Up to this stage, according to Erikson, development mostly depends upon **what is done to** us. From here on out, development depends primarily upon **what we do.** And while adolescence is a stage at which we are neither a child nor an adult,. Life is definitely getting more complex as we attempt to find our own **identity,** struggle with social interactions, and grapple with moral issues. Our task is to discover who we are as individuals separate from our family of origin and as members of a wider society. Unfortunately for those around us, in this process many of us go into a period of withdrawing from responsibilities, which Erikson called a "moratorium." And if we are unsuccessful in navigating this stage, we will experience **role confusion** and upheaval. Those who receive proper encouragement and reinforcement through personal exploration will emerge from this stage with a strong sense of self and a feeling of independence and control. Those who remain unsure of their beliefs and desires will insecure and confused about themselves and the future. A significant task for us is to establish a philosophy of life and in this process we tend to think in terms of ideals, which are conflict free, rather than reality, which is not. The problem is that we don't have much experience and find it easy to substitute ideals for experience. However, we can also develop strong devotion to friends and causes. It is no surprise that our most significant relationships are with peer groups.

Young Adulthood: 18 to 35

Ego development outcome: Intimacy and solidarity vs. isolation

Basic strengths: Affiliation and love

In the initial stage of being an adult we seek one or more companions and love. As we try to find mutually satisfying relationships, primarily through marriage and friends, we generally also begin to start a family, though this age has been pushed back for many couples who today don't start their families until their late thirties. If negotiating this stage is successful, we can experience **intimacy** on a deep level. If we're not successful, **isolation** and distance from others may occur. And when we don't find it easy to create satisfying relationships, our world can begin to shrink as, in defense, we can feel superior to others. Our significant relationships are with marital partners and friends. This stage covers the period of early adulthood when people are exploring personal relationships. Erikson believed it was vital that people develop close, committed relationships with other people. Those who are successful at this step will develop relationships that are committed and secure. Remember that each step builds on skills learned in previous steps. Erikson believed that a strong sense of personal identity was important to developing intimate relationships. Studies have demonstrated that those with a poor sense of self tend to have less committed relationships and are more likely to suffer emotional isolation, loneliness, and depression.

Middle Adulthood: 35 to 55 or 65

Ego development outcome: Generativity vs. self absorption or stagnation

Basic strengths: Production and care

Now work is most crucial. Erikson observed that middle-age is when we tend to be occupied with creative and meaningful work and with issues surrounding our family. The significant task is to perpetuate culture and transmit values of the culture through the family (taming the kids) and working to establish a stable environment. Strength comes through care of others and production of something that contributes to the betterment of society, which Erikson calls **generativity,** so when we're in this stage we often fear inactivity and meaninglessness. As our children leave home, or our relationships or goals change, we may be faced with major life changes-the mid-life crisis-and struggle with finding new meanings and purposes. If we don't get through this stage successfully, we can become **selfabsorbed** and **stagnate.** Significant relationships are within the workplace, the community and the family.

Late Adulthood: 55 or 65 to Death

Ego development outcome: Integrity vs. despair

Basic strengths: Wisdom

This phase occurs during old age and is focused on reflecting back on life. Those who are unsuccessful during this phase will feel that their life has been wasted and will experience many regrets. The individual will be left with feelings of bitterness and despair. Those who feel proud of their accomplishments will feel a sense of integrity. Successfully completing this phase means looking back with few regrets and a general feeling of satisfaction. These individuals will attain wisdom, even when confronting death.

REFLECT YOURSELF

1. Write a short note on psychology of people from infancy to old age.

16

PSYCHOLOGY OF WOMEN, SICK AND CHALLENGED

TOPICS COVERED IN THIS CHAPTER

- Psychology of women, sick and challenged
- Psychology of sick and challenged

PSYCHOLOGY OF WOMEN, SICK AND CHALLENGED

Psychology of Women

The first question which calls for our consideration in this context concerns the functions and duties which a woman can and must discharge, the particular types of psychosynthesis which she can bring about in accordance with her particular psychological constitution, and the many problems which arise from woman's own psyche or in her relation with man. Situations and problems of this nature arise in every woman's life and it is necessary that she face them in a way that is most satisfying to herself and to the other people concerned. The most natural thing and frequent role for woman is that of being man's companion, her wife. An Italian author, Luciod'Ambra, wrote two novels entitled respectively the Occupation of the Husband and the Profession of the Wife. In these different designations an important psychological truth is alluded to, namely that while man's principal functions are his activities outside the family and are of a social character, woman's most important activity, her "profession", is generally in and with the family. To use a less modern but gentle and apt expression: woman is, or should be, "the queen of the home".

Unfortunately, this kingdom of the home is often troubled by silent or noisy disharmonies and conflicts which sometimes shake it to its very foundations and can even dismember it. If we search for the causes of these discords, we discover that there are mainly two: selfishness and lack of understanding. The corresponding remedies can, therefore, be reduced to two principal ones:

The first one is goodness and a spirit of sacrifice. These are hard to develop, but are high qualities which everybody should cultivate because their fruits are most rewarding. The second remedy consists of an intelligent, intuitive, willing psychological and spiritual understanding. This understanding is not easy to acquire because the psychological constitutions of man and woman are deeply different, much more so than we generally realize. One could almost say that they belong to two different species. It therefore seems useful to pause and examine somewhat the differing characteristics of male and female psychology. In speaking frankly, I may at times seem rude to both sexes.

Typically, although by no means universally, there exists between a husband and his wife polarities of psychological functions. The man tends to excel in certain vital operations while the woman manifests others. For example, in dealing with the physical world, man has active, manipulative and creative functions while woman, as wife and mother is primarily concerned with maintaining and preserving the life and resources of the family. On the other hand, in the sphere of the emotions and of the imagination, it is the woman who is usually the better developed, more positive and productive of the two. In this area, the husband is apt to be relatively naive and easily confused. So there is an apparent inversion of dominance functions that man and woman need to appreciate, and therefore collaborate with each other in order to form an effective team.

There is a similar inverted polarity between man and woman in the intellectual sphere. Man tends to be the more rational, logical, and active. He is consciously oriented toward facts, their relationships and their implications. By contrast woman's mental functions are less developed, but balanced by her superiority in another sphere, that of the intuition. This is the capacity for attaining understanding in non-rational and unconscious ways which are fully as valid as man's thoughtful rationality.

These different polarities define some important qualitative distinctions between man and woman. These differences can explain many psychological conflicts and disorders. Speaking of man in general, the average so-called normal man develops qualities and functions such as aggressiveness, mental activity, and efficiency. These he manifests to a marked degree, whereas qualities of a feminine type such as sensitivity, feeling, imagination, and intuition remain in an undeveloped and, at times, almost atrophied conditions. Because these latter functions do not keep pace with the rest of his growth, it therefore often happens that the average man remains relatively primitive and sometimes even barbaric. His imagination, generally repressed in the unconscious, is disordered when it does rise to the surface, and often expresses itself in fancies of which he himself is ashamed. His feeling nature tends to remain primitive; he has neither delicacy nor plasticity. He can pass from outbursts of almost savage passion to hardness and insensitivity, and vice versa, or he can pass from insensibility to almost childish weakness and sentimentality. His intuition is generally rudimentary, almost non-existent. He endeavors to solve all problems, whether practical or abstract, through mental processes only, and because he does not take into consideration the more subtle and imponderable elements, he is often mistaken. In the various events of life, his cleverly formulated plans and programs often come to naught, and instead of finding the faults that lie within himself and his own shortcomings, he blames other people and events for his failures.

The psychological processes of the large majority of women are the very opposite. The average woman's opinion are usually nothing more than prejudices and superstitions to which she clings obstinately, even in the face of factual evidence to the contrary. Of course, her opinions are sometimes correct, especially when based on good intuition, but only too often they are erroneous outcomes of personal emotions, of imaginings of various kinds, or of blindly accepted traditions. It is typical of many women (particularly of those who do not work in the professions or hold executive positions in public life) that they do not consider the true nature of the problems with which they are faced. Their mental activity consists of examining things in an unanalytical, diffuse, and inconclusive manner, with arguments that are often of a personal rather than objective character.

It should therefore be apparent that the one-sided psychological development of the average man or woman engenders deficiencies that result in serious problems. Most men and women are in themselves incomplete, almost psychologically maimed beings. They can find the solution of their problems only through mutual integration, *i.e.*, by combining their qualities so as to constitute together a complete human being.

Man, insofar as his feminine functions are rudimentary, cannot understand and appreciate woman. He feels himself attracted towards her, sometimes irresistibly; vaguely he is aware that she possesses traits he needs, but he does not know how to approach her psychologically. She appears to him as a strange, elusive, chameleon-like creature. The acuity and changeability of her sensitivity, the wealth and plasticity of her imagination disconcert and confound him; her intuition impresses him, but he cannot understand its nature and origin; it perplexes him, and generally he is skeptical concerning it.

The average woman, in her turn, is unable to get out of her subjectivity and personal approach to things, lacks understanding of masculine activities and qualities, and often does not even try to understand them. She loves man, but with a personal, possessive, jealous affection. But although she loves him, she neither understands nor appreciates his world, his interests, his ideals. She is inclined to regard him as a savage who holds a delicate butterfly with a rough hand, who ruthlessly destroys perfumed and many-coloured flowers, as a naughty boy who is inclined to fight with others, as one who foolishly risks his life in darling enterprises, who plays with his complicated machines, and who neglects those who love him in order to chase after ancient ruins or rare manuscripts or to construct difficult and useless theories and systems

PSYCHOLOGY OF SICK AND CHALLENGED

Until recently ideas about the psychology of disability have been exclusively created by non-disabled people and almost always in rehabilitation or medical settings. Generally, these interpreters of the psychology of disability have been able-bodied practitioners (doctors or therapists) who work with disabled adults or, very often, disabled children and their able-bodied parents.

But what is the experience of disability that these 'psychologists' try to interpret?

For most workers, therapists, or psychologists, disability is something that they experience (if I can put it this way) when they walk into a hospital (rehabilitation) ward and stand next to a bed, or enter a physiotherapy or occupational therapy room, and turn their attention onto the problems presented by a 'patient'. Alternatively they might be sitting at their work desks and there is a knock on the door. A disabled person, or parent with a disabled child, comes into the room and a set of problems are presented.

In this experience of disability the problem only appears when the disabled person appears. The worker, therapist, or psychologist, naturally associates the problem with the person because this is the way it is experienced. The workers starts to ask the patient questions which are concerned with the problems that the disabled person may have with dressing, walking, eating, etc. They may substitute observation for questioning but the focus of attention of the professional remains on what the person cannot do, or is having difficulty in doing. The attention is not on *'a functioning disabled person'* living in their own home, at work, or school but, on the contrary, on *'a non-functioning person'* in a medical setting.

Contemporary ideas about the psychology of disability have developed on the basis of three assumptions -(i) disability means you cannot function, *you* have problems (that is why the disabled person is in the medical setting), (ii) disability is something that the individual has, or possesses, it is part of you (you are a *'person with a disability'* you are defined in medical terms; 'disability', here, means a chronic personal impairment) and that is why personal caring services are needed, and (iii) the psychological reactions of the individual are all interpreted in terms of reactions to personal dysfunction.

People with diabetes, blood pressure, cancer, organ failure or aids struggle with these deadly diseases throughout life. They undergo psychological and physical discomfort. They also experience sense of insecurity, pain and all sorts of psychological discomforts. If such people are below poverty line or in low socio-economic status experience more difficulty than the difficulty arising due to their illness. Absence of care taker may worsen the situation.

REFLECT YOURSELF

1. What are the hardships that women, sick and challenged face in society?

17

Psychology of Groups

TOPICS COVERED IN THIS CHAPTER

- GROUP Dynamics

Much of our lives are spent in groups with other people: we form groups to socialise, earn money, play sport, make music, even to change the world. But although groups are diverse, many of the psychological processes involved are remarkably similar.

Group is defined as "two or more persons who are interdependent and share a set of beliefs, values and norms which regulate their mutual conduct for attaining common goals. Kreth and Gruthfield defined it as "a group comes into being to achieve the wants of its members, in the course of interaction the members develop the group ideology which regulates their attitude and actions and influence their satisfaction." According to T.M. Newton, group consists of two or more persons who share norms about certain things with one another and whose social roles are closely interlocked." Whereas, crowd is a collection of individuals who are all attending and reacting to some common objects, their reactions being of simple pre-potent sort and accompanied by strong emotional responses", as defined by F. Allport. Group has a common goal to pursue. In a crowd there is no common goal. Groups have a group ideology and a group structure. Members have differentiated roles whereas, in a crowd there is no common ideology and crowd is highly unstructured. The term role is absent in the latter. Group behaviour is rational in nature and involves well thought out plan of action whereas, crowd behaviour is irrational in nature and does not involve well thought out plan of action. Group members have a strong sense of belongingness whereas, crowd lack the sense of belongingness. Group is a relatively more stable than a crowd. Group functions according to a set of rules or norms whereas, crowd activities do not confirm to the norms of the expected behaviour. Group formation may either deliberate or spontaneous, whereas, crowd can be of a causal one like audience or aggressive one like a mob.

GROUP DYNAMICS

1. **Groups formation:** The desire to form and join social groups is extremely powerful and built into our nature. Amongst other things groups give us a most valuable gift, our social identity, which contributes to our sense of who we are. Just how readily people form and join groups is demonstrated by Tajfel etal. (1971) in the so-called 'minimal groups paradigm'. In their study boys who were strangers to each other were given only the slightest hint that they they were being split into two groups. Even without knowing or seeing who else was in their group they favoured members of their own group over the others. Group behaviour, then, can arise from almost nothing. There is an objective which is accepted by most of its members as the group goal. Members who are greatly influenced by the ideas of attaining group goal experience feelings of group belongingness. People join groups because group-goal satisfies their wants. So, different people having various needs work together. We categorize such a group in terms of their major group goals like religious organizations. If such a group continue to exist over a period of time, it often acquires accessory goals. for example, religious organizations work upon educational goal expanded to health services further, to community service.
2. **Initiation rites improve group evaluations:** Existing groups don't let others join for free: the cost is sometimes monetary, sometimes intellectual, sometimes physical-but usually there is an initiation rite. So, not only do groups want to test you, but they want you to value your membership.
3. **Groups breed conformity:** After joining a group and being initiated, we have to get a feel for the group norms, the rules of behaviour in that group. Group norms can be extremely powerful, bending our behaviours in ways we would never expect.

   One of the most famous experiments showing how easily we conform to unwritten group rules was conducted by Asch (1951). He had participants sit amongst a group of other people, judging the length of a line. The trick was that all the other members of the group were confederates of the experimenter who had been told to lie about which line was longer. Incredibly 76% of participants denied the evidence from their own senses at least once, just to conform with the group. Afterwards people made up all kinds of excuses for their behaviour. Most popular was a variation on: "that many people can't be wrong". Oh yes they can.
4. **Learn the ropes or be ostracised:** Group norms are extremely pervasive: this becomes all the more obvious when we start breaking them. Break the group's rules and you'll know about it soon enough.

   Although groups have norms-rules that apply to everyone in the group-people have roles within groups and corresponding rules that apply to just their position. All the group members share common beliefs, values, ideas and common norms known as group ideology. Beliefs refer to set of ideas, knowledge relevant to common goals of the group members. Values reflect group goals. they refer to beliefs about what objects and actions are good and desirable. The norms or rules of behaviour are laid so that group functions smoothly in a disciplined manner, by specifying rewards for adherence and punishment for non-adherance.
5. **Leaders gain trust by conforming:** A high-profile, high-status role in any group is that of its leader, but where do leaders come from? In some groups, they are appointed or imposed from outside, but in many groups leaders emerge slowly and subtly from the ranks.

A study that has much to teach was carried out by Merei (1949) who observed children at a Hungarian nursery school. He noticed that successful leaders were those who initially fitted in with the group then slowly began to suggest new activities adapted from the old. Children didn't follow potential leaders who jumped straight in with new ideas. Leaders first conform, then only later, when trust has been gained, can they be confident that others will follow.

6. **Groups can improve performance ... known as social facilitation:** The mere presence of others can make us perform better. Social psychology pioneer Norman Triplett noticed that racing cyclists with a pacemaker covered each mile about 5 seconds quicker than those without (Triplett, 1898). Later research found this wasn't *all* about the effects of competition. The presence of other people seems to facilitate our own performance, but more so when the task is relatively separate to others and can be judged on its own merits. This phenomenon is called Social Facilitation (Guerin, 1993), and as we try harder due to the presence of others, our performance actually decreases for difficult or unlearned tasks. Think about learning to play basketball for the first time. If you are alone, you will likely be more relaxed, and better able to concentrate. When others are watching you, however, you are more likely to be self-conscious, and therefore make more mistakes. Professional basketball players, however, because the task is so well learned, perform better when others are watching and they are able demonstrate their confidence and ability.
7. **Social loafing:** In other circumstances, though, people in groups demonstrate a tremendous capacity for loafing. Another social psychology pioneer, Max Ringelmann, found in the 1890s that participants in a tug 'of war only put in half as much effort when they were in a team of 8 than when they were on their own. It seems that when hiding in the group is easy, for example when tasks are additive and each person's contribution is difficult to judge, people will slack off to an impressive degree.
8. **The grapevine is 80% accurate:** Intelligence, rumour, gossip and tittle-tattle is the lifeblood of many groups. It travels at a tremendous pace in big organisations because people love a good bit of gossip, but what are 'they' talking about and can you believe what 'they' say?
9. **Groups breed competition-concept of we groups and they group/ingroup and outgroup:** While co-operation *within* group members is generally not so much of a problem, co-operation *between* groups can be hellish. People may be individually co-operative, but once put in a 'them-and-us' situation, rapidly become remarkably adversarial.

   Insko et. al. (2001) had participants playing a classic game called 'the prisoner's dilemma' which they used to measure competitiveness. When on their own people were competitive 37%.of the time but when they were in a group of three this increased to 54%. People easily become suspicious of other groups, reasoning that while their individual members may be 'alright', the group as a whole cannot be trusted. Group members perceive each other as belonging to whole or unit. They have the consciousness of group belonging.
10. **Group Think and Group Polarization:** If you've ever been involved in a group decision making process, you've probably seen one of two things happen: either the group agrees on all of the major issues, or there is significant dissent that splits the group. If the group is cohesive; if they agree on most issues, they tend to stifle dissent because group harmony is the anticipated outcome (Janis, 1972). When we all agree, and are happy with that agreement,

we typically do not want to hear opposing arguments. This phenomenon is referred to as **Group Think.** It can lead to impulsive decisions and a failure to identify and! or consider all sides of an argument.

Similar to this, **Group Polarization** refers to a groups tendency to talk itself into extreme positions. In this case, a group gets so focused and energized about a decision that it creates an internal fuel, so to speak, which pushes itself forward faster than originally intended. Imagine a group of protesters, all agreeing and deciding to picket. You can see how this could get out of hand because opposing views (Group Think) are not considered and the push to move forward for the cause is fueled internally (Group Polarization).

11. **Bystander Effect:** This last phenomenon is an unfortunate reality which has been observed far to many times in groups and in larger cities. We've all heard stories of people getting mugged, or beaten, or raped in broad daylight while people around offered no assistance. We have found that the internal push to help a person in need decreases as the group gets larger, very similar to Social Loafing. In this instance, however, people tend to be followers and will only get involved if they witness another person getting involved. What results is a group of people witnessing a crime and wondering why nobody is helping. This does not occur if you are the only person witnessing the crime. If nobody else is around, a person will tend to help the victim. The more people, however, the less likely someone will offer assistance.
12. **Why Group Norms Kill Creativity: Research shows group members equate creativity with conformity.** Creativity is a much coveted asset for a very simple reason: an idea that transcends orthodoxy has the power to bring wealth, fame and status. Commercial, scientific, educational and artistic organisations, therefore, often talk about how they want to foster creativity.

Unfortunately groups only rarely fragment great ideas because people in them are powerfully shaped by group norms: the unwritten rules which describe how individuals in a group 'are' and how they 'ought' to behave. These unwritten rules or 'groups norms' flow almost imperceptibly from one person to the next so that changes are difficult to spot unless they are carefully measured. A classic psychological study on group norms randomly allocated new university students to either conservative sororities or more liberal dormitories (Siegel and Siegel, 1957). Over time students assigned to the liberal dormitories became less conservative as the group's norms seeped into their consciousness.

Not only do norms spread like wildfire, groups don't even need to be that well-established, people will conform to others with only the slightest encouragement. In another classic social psychology study people thrown into a group of strangers denied their own senses to increase their conformity with others. When simply judging the length of a line, participants happily went along with the group despite clear evidence from their eyes that the group was wrong.

The purpose of norms is to provide a stable and predictable social world, to regulate our behaviour with each other. In many respects norms have a beneficial effect, bolstering society's foundations and keeping it from falling into chaos. On the other hand stability and predictability are enemies of the creative process. When groups are asked to think creatively the reason they frequently fail is because implicit norms constrain them in the most explicit ways. This is clearly demonstrated in a recent study carried out by Adarves-Y orno et al. (2006). They asked two groups of participants to create posters and subtly gave each group a norm about either using more words on the poster or more images. Afterwards when they judged each others' work, participants equated creativity with following the group norm; the 'words' group rated posters with more words as more creative and the 'images' group rated posters with more images as more creative. The unwritten rules of the group, therefore, determined what its members considered creative. In effect groups had redefined creativity as conformity. In another part of the same experiment these results were reversed when people's individuality rather than their group membership was emphasised. Creativity became all about being different from others and being inconsistent with group norms. When freed from the almost invisible shackles of the group, then, people suddenly remembered the dictionary definition of creativity: to transcend the orthodox.

REFLECT YOURSELF

1. Discuss the group dynamics.

18

Mental Hygiene and Mental Health

TOPICS COVERED IN THIS CHAPTER

- Mental Hygiene and Mental Health
- Characteristics of Mentally Healthy Person
- What are the Warning Signs of Mental Illness?
- Promotive and Preventive Mental Health Strategies and Services
- Guidance and Counselling

MENTAL HYGIENE AND MENTAL HEALTH

Concept of Mental Health

A healthy individual is not only physically healthy, but is also mentally healthy. Health is a state of being hale, sound or whole, in body, mind or soul. It means that both body and mind are working efficiently and harmoniously. It includes a sound, efficient mind and controlled emotions. Mental health which today is recognized as an important aspect of one's total health status. John, Sutton and Webster defined it as a positive but relative quality of life. It is a condition which is characteristic of the average person who meets the demands of life on the basis of his own capacities and limitations. By 'relative' we mean the degree of mental health which an individual enjoys at a time is continuously changing. It is not mere absence of mental illness that constitutes mental health. On the other hand, it is a positive, active quality of the individual's daily living. It means the ability to balance feelings, desires, ambitions and ideals in one's daily living. It means the ability to face and accept realities of life. It connotes such habits of work and attitudes towards people and things that bring maximum satisfaction and happiness to the individual. Mental health has two aspects, individual and social. Individual aspect means that he/she is skilful to be able to adapt to new situations. He/she is self confident, adequate and free from internal conflicts or inconsistencies. But he achieves this internal adjustment in a social set up. Society has value systems, customs and traditions by which it governs itself and promotes the general welfare of its members. It is within this social framework that the internal adjustment has to be built up.

Concept of Mental Hygiene

Mental hygiene deals with principles of living which would serve as a guide to human adjustments. Mental hygiene is an organized attempt to effect human adjustment through the application of these few principles and practices. It has three major purposes:

(a) The prevention of mental disorders
(b) Preservation of mental health of the individual and group
(c) Discovery and utilization of therapeutic measures to cure mental illness.

CHARACTERISTICS OF A MENTALLY HEALTHY PERSON

1. A mentally healthy person is aware of his motives, desires, weaknesses and strengths.
2. He has a sense of personal worth, self-respect and feels secure in a group.
3. He feels that he is wanted or loved.
4. He has faith in his ability to succeed whatever he undertakes.
5. He can get along with other people.
6. He has understanding of his environment, does not fear future.
7. He does not evade responsibility or duty.
8. A mentally healthy person lives in reality and not in fantasy.
9. He has developed a capacity to tolerate frustrations and disappointments in his daily life. He is able to regulate his emotions in a socially desirable manner.
10. He practices good health habits such as sleep, rest, nutrition, physical activity, personal cleanliness and protection from disease.
11. He is able to think on own and take decisions.
12. He has the ability to get enjoyment and satisfaction out of his daily routine job.

WHAT ARE THE WARNING SIGNS OF MENTAL ILLNESS?

In an **adult**: A person with one or more of the following symptoms should be evaluated by a psychiatrist or other physician as soon as possible:

- Marked personality change
- Inability to cope with problems and daily activities
- Strange or grandiose ideas.
- Excessive anxieties.
- Prolonged depression and apathy.
- Marked changes in eating or sleeping patterns.
- Extreme highs and lows.
- Abuse of alcohol or drugs.
- Excessive anger, hostility, or violent behaviour.
- A person who is thinking or talking about suicide or homicide should seek help immediately.
- Confused thinking

- Long-lasting sadness or irritability

  In a **child:** Having only one or two of the problems listed below is not necessarily cause for alarm. They may simply indicate that a practical solution is called for, such as more consistent discipline or a visit with the child's teachers or guidance counselor to see whether there is anything out of the ordinary going on at school. A combination of symptoms, however, is a signal for professional intervention.
- The child seems overwhelmed and troubled by his or her feelings, unable to cope with them.
- The child cries a lot.
- The child frequently asks or hints for help.
- The child seems constantly preoccupied, worried, anxious, and intense. Some children develop a fear of a variety of things—rain, barking dogs, burglars, their parents' getting killed when out of sight, and so on—while other children simply wear their anxiety on their faces.
- The child has fears or phobias that are unreasonable or interfere with normal activities.
- The child can't seem to concentrate on schoolwork and other age-appropriate tasks.
- The child's school performance declines and doesn't pick up again.
- The child's teachers, school administrators, or other authority figures in the child's life ask the parent what might be troubling the child.
- The child is having difficulty mastering school work.
- Teachers suggest that the child may have a learning disability or other type of school related problem.
- The child loses interest in playing.
- The child tries to stimulate himself or herself in various ways. Examples of this kind of behaviour include excessive thumb sucking or hair pulling, rocking of the body, head banging to the point of hurting himself, and masturbating often or in public.
- The child has no friends and gets into fights with other youngsters. Teachers or others may report that "this is a very angry or disruptive kid."
- The child isolates himself or herself from other people.
- The child regularly talks about death and dying.
- The child appears to have low self-esteem and little self—confidence. Over and over the child may make such comments as: "I can't do anything right." "I'm so stupid." "I don't see why anyone would love me." "I know you [or someone else] hates me." "Nobody likes me." "I'm ugly ... too big ... too small. ..too fat. .. too skinny ... too tall. .. too short, etc."
- Sleep difficulties don't appear to be resolving. They include refusing to be separated from one or both parents at bedtime, inability to sleep, sleeping too much, sleeping on parents' bed, nightmares, and night terrors.
- The child begins to act in a provocatively sexual manner, This is more common in girls as they approach puberty and thereafter, but even much younger girls may flirt with men in sexually suggestive ways.
- The child sets fires.
- Some symptoms or reactions are so serious that a pediatrician or a psychiatrist should be consulted **immediately:**
- The child appears to be accident prone. In younger children a succession of accidents can become the equivalent of suicide attempts.

- The child mutilates himself in some way—cutting or scarring himself, pulling out his hair, or biting fingernails until nail beds bleed.
- The child mutilates or kills animals.
- The child's eating habits change to the point that his weight is affected. This can be caused by either overeating or undereating.
- The child adopts ritualistic behaviours. This is indicative of obsessive-compulsive disorder, A child may have to line up her toys in a certain way every night, for example, or get ready for bed following a routine that never varies. If she forgets one item in the routine, she must start all over again.
- The child beats up others—another child, a parent, or other adult.
- The child is using alcohol or other drugs.
- The child is sexually active or on the verge of becoming so. Again, this is rare in children 12 and under but certainly not unheard of, especially since there is great pressure on kids today to become sexually active at progressively earlier ages.

PROMOTIVE AND PREVENTIVE MENTAL HEALTH STRATEGIES AND SERVICES

Promotion of Mental Health

- WHO defines health promotion as *"the process of enabling people to increase control over, and to improve their health"* (WHO, 1986). Mental health promotion often refers to positive mental health, rather than mental ill health. Positive mental health is the desired outcome of health promotion interventions. *Mental health promotion* is any action taken to maximize mental health and well being among populations and individuals (Commonwealth Department of Health and Aged Care, 2000).

  Objectives and Actions of Mental Health Promotion: Health promotion is an approach to improving public health that requires broad participation. Mental health promotion is an integral part of health promotion theory and practice. The personal, social and environmental factors that determine mental health and mental illness may be clustered conceptually around three themes
- *The development and maintenance of healthy communities:* This provides a safe and secure environment, good housing, positive educational experiences, employment, good working conditions and a supportive political infrastructure; minimizes conflict and violence; allows self-determination and control of one's life; and provides community validation, social support, positive role models and the basic needs of food, warmth and shelter.

Each person's ability to deal with the social world through skills like participating, tolerating diversity and mutual responsibility. This is associated with positive experiences of early bonding, attachment, relationships, communication and feelings of acceptance.

Each person's ability to deal with thoughts and feelings, the management of life and emotional resilience

This is associated with self-esteem, the ability to manage conflict and the ability to learn.

- Health promotion and prevention are necessarily related and overlapping activities:
- The former is concerned with the determinants of health and the latter focuses on the causes of disease. The evidence for prevention of mental disorders contributes to the evidence for the promotion of mental health.

- The actions that promote mental health will often have as an important outcome the prevention of mental disorders.

There are different organizations at state level or world level that use both preventive and promotive strategies to combat mental diseases. Let's see one of India's best treatment centre of mental disorders is NIMHANS.

Services provided by NIMHANS: Following services are provided:

- Psychosocial study of the patients and their families.
- Home visits for diagnostic and therapeutic services.
- Community agencies contacts for Resource mobilization.
- Educating the patients/family members about the illnesses, treatment and rehabilitation.
- Marital counseling/therapy/intervention services.
- Family counseling/therapy/intervention services.
- Group interaction/intervention services for patients/family members.
- Liaison services with families and community.
- Training the para—professionals and non-professionals in mental health services.
- Extension services—camps and outreach programmes.

These services are offered in various permutations and combinations depending on the nature of the problems, felt needs of the patients, families and communities. In addition to the therapeutic or treatment services, certain promotive/preventive services are also undertaken by the members of the Department in collaboration with voluntary agencies, factories, educational institutions etc.

Mission Statement of NIMHANS

- To provide the best possible psychosocial services for the persons affected with psychiatric, neurological and neuro-surgical problems by involving the inherent potentials in the clients, families and communities.
- To offer advanced level of teaching and training in psychiatric social work.
- To undertake socially relevant and culturally appropriate researches to help understand, assess and develop cost effective psychosocial intervention 'strategies.
- To Enrich the collaboration and co-operation with Schools of Social Work/Post Graduate Department of Social Work and other Governmental and Non-governmental organisations related to health, education, welfare and developmental Institutions.
- To formulate appropriate policies involving psychiatric social work ingredients for the promotion of mental health, prevention, treatment and rehabilitation of mental health problems.

  Preventive mental health strategies: "To prevent" literally means "to keep something from happening". However, there are different notions about that "something" and they have been identified as the incidence of a disorder, its relapses, the disability associated with it, or the risks for a disorder-and this has led to confusion in the field of mental health regarding the term prevention (Mrazek and Haggerty, 1994).

  Historically, the public health concept of disease prevention has viewed prevention as *primary, secondary or tertiary* depending on whether the strategy prevents the disease itself, the severity of the disease or the associated disability.

  The following three categories of *primary prevention* have been identified:

- *Universal prevention*: targeting the general public or a whole population group.
- *Selective prevention*: targeting individuals or subgroups of the population whose risk of developing a mental disorder is significantly higher than that of the rest of the population.
- *Indicated prevention*: targeting persons at high-risk for mental disorders.

  Secondary prevention refers to interventions undertaken to reduce the prevalence, i.e., all specific treatment-related strategies, and *tertiary prevention* would include interventions that reduce disability and all forms of rehabilitation as well as prevention of relapses of the illness.
- The National Mental Health Programme serves practically as the mental health policy. There was an eight-fold increase in budget allocation for the National Mental Health Programme for the Tenth Five-Year Plan (2002–2007).

Mental Health Services

Mental Health Services in a community are a concern not only with early diagnosis and treatment but also preservation and promotion of good mental health and prevention of mental illness.

Mental Health Services Comprise of:

1. Early diagnosis and treatment
2. Rehabilitation
3. Group and individual psychotherapy
4. Mental health education
5. Use of modem psychoactive drugs
6. After care services.

Comprehensive Mental Health Programme

Community Mental Health Programme consist of:

1. In-patient services
2. Out-patient services
3. Partial hospitalisation
4. Emergency services
5. Diagnostic services
6. Pre-care and aftercare services including home
7. Education services
8. Training
9. Research and evaluation.

GUIDANCE AND COUNSELLING

Concept of Guidance

Guidance has been defined as the process of assisting the students in their education, vocational and social development. The term 'guidance' derives its meaning from the word guide which means to direct or to lead. To guide, implies the act of giving the needed information regarding places, problems, subjects, situations or individuals. Henix Erickson defined it as "guidance is helping the students to become adjusted to its present situation and to plan his future in lying with his interest and abilities and social needs." Generally guidance is defined in accordance with social context as "a process of helping each individual to help oneself to recognize and use one's inner resources to set goals, make plans, and work out one's own problems of development under the most favourable conditions that society can provide". Gilbert Wren and Wills Dugan have some special principles of guidance. These are:

1. It is concerned with the whole student not various intellectual aspects of life.
2. Guidance is concerned with all students and not with special or problem children.
3. It is concerned primarily with prevention rather than cure.
4. It is more than the activity of a specialist involves whole school staff.
5. It is a continous process which goes on throughout the school life of a student.

Through a guidance programme a student is assisted to:

- Understand himself
- Make use of his/her most of the abilities
- Develop the ability of making wise choices, decision making independently.
- Adjust himself to varied situations.
- Make unique contribution to the society.

The present day concept of guidance is used synonymously with the term education, as an all round development of a student. Guidance service comprise of collecting information about vocational, educational personal opportunities so that individual makes realistic choices and decisions.

Concept of Counselling

The term "counselling" derives its meaning from the word counsel which means to give advice, consultation, opinion or suggestion. Counselling has been defined as a face to face relationship between a trained counsellor and a counsellee , which is seeking help in gaining self-understanding, decision making and skills for problem-solving. E.G. Vedanayagam defined counselling "as an accepting, trusting and safe relationship in which clients learn to define their goals, to acquire the essential social skills and to develop the courage and self confidence to implement desired new behaviour". Counselling is the central activity of the guidance service where a trained counsellor with lot of acumen, technical knowledge, effective communication, empathy, honesty and acceptance, trust, patience and experience assist the counsellee in—helping to increase self understanding, self-realization and self-acceptance, --decision making by

(a) Providing situation to affect change in behaviour
(b) Utilizing peer consensus to affect behaviour
(c) Using behaviour modifications procedure by giving proper reinforcement to bring about behavioural change.

Relationship between Guidance and Counselling

Guidance is a systematic and organized service designed to meet the individual needs of all the students in schools. Detailed information about all students is collected, recorded and interpreted.

It helps to identify and develop the abilities and interests of students. Students are also given information about educational and vocational opportunities open to them and are helped in career planning and selection. While helping students in their all-round development it is observed that some students need individual attention in solving their problems. Family members, school teachers help such students to solve their problems. But a trained counsellor or a specialist is required as through their technical knowledge and experience are able to deal such problems of individuals more effectively. Thus, a face to face relationship between a trained counsellor and a counsellee who is seeking a help in gaining self understanding , self acceptance and self-realization , decision making and skills for problem solving referred to as counselling. Here an individual is treated as a unique person in a unique situation.

Some of the guidance work like collecting career information, individual student can be done by any guidance worker. But actual assistance can be given through counselling as it requires a high level of skill as well as professional training.

Thus, both the terms are mutually related but not are synonymous.

Difference between Guidance and Counselling

- Guidance can be given to a large group of individuals. It is given before in hand as it is concerned primarily with prevention than cure. Guidance is a long term process for example it goes on throughout school life.
- Counseling can be done to a single individual where a specific problem is solved. It is given only when a particular problem arises and inhibits the goals of the individual and such individuals are not able to deal with. Counselling requires a high level of skill as well as special professional training with technical knowledge whereas it is not required in guidance. Whereas, counselling is being a professional consultation is a short term process, where it ends when the problem of the client or counsellee gets solved.

NOTE: Today's nurse is living in a fast changing world with all its technological achievements: with the mechanization and urbanization of society, her working conditions are rapidly changing. The nurse has to deal with different people having different problems both physically and mentally. To serve them satisfactory, a knowledge of human psychology is essential. Nursing is a profession which follows a uniform standard of training for nurses and midwives established by Indian Nursing Council in India. It is an autonomous body under the Government of India, Ministry of Health and Family Welfare. It is a skilled discipline which helps to improve the overall health status of individuals, groups and communities. It is a profession which focuses upon not only the promotive but also preventive health services. It covers all aspects related to disease but also in supporting people during illness, recovery and rehabilitation. It is a profession which involves helping and caring by applying intellectual, interpersonal and technical skills. Nursing is a diverse profession which covers nursing for children, adults, mental health nursing and nursing for people with learning disability.

REFLECT YOURSELF

1. Elucidate upon differences between guidance and counselling.
2. Write a short note on mental hygiene.
3. Write a short note on warning signs of mental illness.

19

PSYCHOLOGY AND ITS RELEVANCE TO NURSING

TOPICS COVERED IN THIS CHAPTER

INTRODUCTION

Psychology is study of behaviour both animal and human behaviour. It is also a study of both overt and covert behaviour. A patient is a person who is stress due to physical condition or mental condition and cannot treat this situation on his own. He requires doctor and a nurse to treat him. Here comes the play of a nurse who is a facilitator in the process of healing. Let's discover the personality traits of a nurse and interaction of psychology with nursing.

PERSONALITY TRAITS OF A NURSE

- Nurse should be in discipline.
- He/she should be a responsible person as they provide care.
- Nurse should be patient during absence of a doctor.
- Nursing profession demands commitment, dedication and punctuality.
- It is a profession which works on toes i.e., hardwork.
- Just like hospitality industry, nurses should have good physical stamina, alertness of mind and adaptability to follow tough working schedules.
- Nurse should be calm, pleasant and equipped with good communication skill.

DUTIES OF A NURSE

- Being a patient advocate when the patient themselves cannot because of illness or lack of proper health knowledge.
- Being a patient educator by explaining procedures and treatments. For instance, nurses take care that patient takes medicines, change wound dressings, and knows the use of health care equipment.
- Supporting the patient in time of need.
- Educating people about how to take preventive steps in catching up transmittable disease, violence, obesity and tobacco use also maternal child education.
- Nurses also take up higher education such as masters or Phd degrees in nursing. They may work as policy makers, managers, educators and scholars. A nurse trained in educational psychology can be an effective health educator to explain to the patient and the relatives:'
    - The nature and diagnostic examination, findings and treatment.
    - Principles of health and prevention of diseases
    - After care programmes and rehabilitation
- A good understanding of the patient by the nurse can be the best social support to patients who are hospitalized and also while coping with chronic mental illness.
- An infant is in the need of tender loving care in the hospital. Touching the infant is the first communication from the nurse. She should plan to give as much personal attention as possible such as cuddling, handling etc. An accurate observation is imp. As it cannot speak. She must.be able to interpret the infant's needs through its crying and it's body language. She should observe the physical abnormalities and unusually growth and development. Assisting, teaching and advising the mother is the responsibility of the nurse. New mothers need emotional support and encouragement.
- The older child is gaining more independence but continues to need guidance and special care. He needs direction to understand what behaviour is expected of him or what are the do's and don'ts when hospitalized. The child needs frequent praise and encouragement especially in loneliness, pain and discomfort.
- The elderly need warmth and personal touch of others and should be helped to prevent social isolation. They have a special need to be respected and valued as a person. The nurse should help the elderly hear and see more easily. They should be physically protected if they are disoriented.
- Old people become impatient and show irritability and willfulness. She should realize that these are due to the normal deteriorating process. It is necessary to keep them interested in life and make them feel important and useful.
- The nurse should always be aware of the need for the satisfaction of the primary needs such as proper food and constant supply of air or oxygen should be met.
- Patient on admission to the ward does not know the do's and don't's in the ward. She must introduce himself as the nurse concerned with his care and give him a general geography of the ward with which the patient can quickly become familiar also will add to security.
- Nurse should restrain "talking down" to patients when giving instructions or information. She should avoid intrusive history taking and should keep all information strictly confidential.

RELATIONSHIP BETWEEN PSYCHOLOGY AND NURSING

- Nurses who know the psychological concepts, may apply in their relative field. Such as understanding diverse patient's needs as patient's differ in characteristics and behaviour.
- Nurses may also understand their own needs, motives and behaviour which may help in giving care to the patient because in the hospital there are patients, at home, there are people who need care. In the community health nursing field, there are people of all ages who need to educated and also other members of the health team.
- It will help her to improve situations by helping others solve problems.
- Nurse recognizes her own emotions which affect her body and she will recognize the same in her patients.
- Not only how to deal with psychological concepts, nurses are also asked to perform psychometric assessments either in absence of a clinical psychologist or assisting them. This happens widely in child development centre.
- The interrelationship of the body, mind and everything happening to the person is extremely important in nursing care. It is necessary to study a person's entire physical and psychological situation to provide him the most helpful nursing care.
- The nurse must be aware of the power of the unconsciousness in her as well as her patient's behaviour. Patients may have unexplained fear of hospitalization or laboratory procedures.
- The work of a nurse in the classrooms and the clinics involve accurate observation. A nurse has to feel the pulse, read the thermometer, record readings on charts, note any changes in the patient conditions, follow instructions and administer doses of medicine to the patient. In all these activities, she has to be absolutely accurate.
- Observation involves two mental activities —attention and perception
- Accurate perception and observation are advantageous for the nurse. Some positive results are accurate learning, adjusting more quickly, good judgement, better memory, more helpful and effective nursing care, improved recording and reporting resulting in fewer accidents and growing personal confidence.
- Particular attention must be given to a patient with any defect in vision or hearing, those who are only partially aware of their environment because of sedation makes it difficult to observe what is going on. Demonstrating and allowing the patient to touch, confirming the pt's perception when he is right and correcting him when he is mistaken are essential to good nursing.
- Understanding defense mechanism will enable the nurse to support the patient and his family. Denial is a reaction to a serious diagnosis or at the time of death. The patient and his family should be allowed to deny the situation until they are prepared to face the reality. The patient will often practice regression through tears, trembling or demanding special treatment.
- Identification can be seen in patient's who rely heavily on the nurse's advice and support. They expect that all of their needs will be met. This can be used constructively to teach proper health care.
- Patients who deal with the stress of serious illness may shift the blame for their condition onto the nurse. They may complain of poor nursing care. She should not show anger and retaliate but should encourage the patients to explore the realistic aspects of their situation.

- The nurse who carries out an assessment of a new patient may be prevented from giving an adequate history by his attitude to his illness. She who attempts to assess the patient's attitude in order to plan appropriate care, herself brings into the situation her own complex attitude system. Her previous nursing experiences influences her attitude towards hospital's staff, treatment and patients. She needs to develop and cultivate professional attitude which will contribute to her success in her work.
- She should try to understand her patient's attitudes. They may have favorable or unfavorable attitude due to their own previous experience.
- The nurse should try to find out the cause of unfavorable attitudes and should change them into favorable ones, because favorable attitudes help in treatment and recovery. She can do this by providing better experience, by adequate explanations, by giving them a feeling of security and self confidence, by means of efficient and skillful care, assurances and giving them sense of being at peace.
- Nursing requires a certain number of special aptitudes. Manual dexterity is useful in practical bedside nursing: speed is useful in all nursing tasks. Linguistic ability makes exam easier. Special aptitudes in sports, music or art may be of great value to psychiatric nurses in the rehabilitation of patients.
- A knowledge of the aptitudes, their measurement and conditions will be helpful to the nurse to develop a proper a aptitude for her profession and to guide those around her. This will also give her an optimism in her own future success.
- The study of educational psychology will help the student nurse to study more effectively, improve her memory and understand the individual differences between nursing students. With understanding her capacity she can plan her academic achievements.
- It will also help her understand and to develop positive attitudes towards patients and problems of other people and in accepting newer technology.
- It would prepare them to be future teachers, understanding the students and their problems and teach more effectively with a better understanding of the advancements in educational technology.
- Knowledge of intellectual functioning is useful to a student nurse and later on for her as a teacher. Assessment and understanding of intellectual functions will be helpful to the nurse in her clinical work. Understanding the development of intelligence in babies and children is another challenge for the nurse.
- Nursing practice is improved by an ability to think creatively and use reliable problem solving methods. The nurse can practice good habits of thinking and systematic problem solving in the profession and all areas of her life like planning her career, difficulty in professional relationships.
- Daily problem solving is a major challenge for the nurse. It is important to have accurate data upon which to base reasoning or problem solving. Much of the data will be gathered through observation and perception. Other data may be supplied through monitors, lab tests and other members of the health team.
- The knowledge of the motivation process will help the nurse in her profession as follows:
  - Help her in maintaining her own mental health
  - Be helpful in her adjustment with patient and relatives

- Will give her an etiology of patients behaviour leading to better to understanding.
- Will help her in the diagnosing of the disease.
- Will facilitate faster cure of the disease.
- Will give her job satisfaction.
- Will be useful in solving most of the problems in interpersonal relationships
- Will improve her relations with her colleagues.

COPING WITH STRESS

Since nursing profession requires commitment, therefore coping with stress becomes an important issue. A nurse by being punctual, planning the daily programme, arranging the study environment and developing the basic abilities with motivation, prompt warming up everyday. Nurse should be able to develop a positive attitude even in handling cases which may turn up disappointing. Balance your life activities with work and play, family and friends and time for self. A nurse can meditate to promote relaxation, slow down pace of life, organize her life with priorities so that she will always accomplish what must be done at the right time, develop healthy social relationships and understand and accept what she can and what she cannot do.

REFLECT YOURSELF

1. Write a short note on the interaction of psychology with nursing.

SECTION-II

Practical

20

INTRODUCTION TO EXPERIMENTAL METHOD

TOPICS COVERED IN THIS CHAPTER

- Definition
- Types of Experiment
- Variables
- Scheme of Psychological Experiment
- Types of Experimental Design
- Advantages and Limitations of Experimental Method
- Application of Experimental Methods in other Branches of Psychology

DEFINITION

Experimental psychology is a separate field of scientific inquiry. Brenato, Binet, James, Watson, Titchener and Skinner were some of the best known shapers of experimental psychology. There are several characteristics of experimental psychology. The experiment starts with some purpose in mind. He knows what selected aspects of behaviour to observe and when to observe them. Experimenter (Er) creates his own opportunities to measure and record behaviour. Moreover, he controls the events under best possible condition, also he can repeat the events and thus obtain idea of how consistent is the phenomenon he is studying. The experimenter can specify his procedure so that both he and others can repeat the process. Having control of the conditions, the experimenter can usually manipulate them systematically to the end that he can specify the effects on behaviour of making certain changes in the condition.

TYPES OF EXPERIMENT

Qualitative and Quantitative

Qualitative experiments are experiments where results are expressed as good or bad or satisfactory. Quantitative experiments are experiments where results are expressed in units or which have numeric value.

Exploratory and Confirmatory

"I wonder what would happen if I did this" type of questions are asked in exploratory experiments and "I'll bet this would happen if I did this" type of questions are the content of confirmatory experiments. In early development of science, many of the experiment are the result of the I wonder what would happen if I did this type of question seeking to know whether or not the factor in question is an effective stimulus variable *i.e.,* will it influence the response? As more facts are accumulated with a science the I wonder what would happen type of problem gives way to what we may call the I'll bet this would happen if I did this type. In this case the experimenter has already certain facts and from the implications of those facts he decides or deduces that if he performed another experiment of a certain nature the results would be such and such *i.e.,* there were confirmatory in sense.

Today psychology is getting well launched into this I'll bet this would happen stage.

VARIABLES

Any particular observation is called a value of the variable. For instance, for the face of a coin there are only two possible values of the variable. Heads or tails, the value of a variable indicates the class to which an observation is to be assigned. By variable we mean anything which we can observe *i.e.,* of such a nature that each single observation can be classified into one and only one of a number of mutually exclusive classes. Variables have to be assessed in an objective manner so that investigation can be repeated and verified by others. Occasionally a variable is solved to classes or categories as boys and girls separated for sex differences. Sometimes variables are subject to ordinary physical measurement. For example, hours of sleep deprivation. Also sometimes, variables have to be scaled in a manner that places them in sort of an order. For example, a psychotherapist might use a five point scale. For purposes of precise communication numbers are assigned to variables.

Types of Variables

Stimulus variable

The general class of things which we observe and relate to the environment, situations or conditions of stimulation is referred to stimulus variables. The stimulus variable in a psychological experiment may consist of electric shock, light, sound, pressure which may be quantified by measuring the physical intensity of stimulus. There are other variables which cannot be quantified such as — problem solving situation, motor conflict situations, social situation.

Behavioural variables

We mean any variable that refers to some action or response of an organism. At one extreme, these actions may consist of relatively simple responses such as finger flexions, eye blink, marking true or false for an item on a test. At other extreme we have complex behaviour patterns as those involved in problem-solving, type writing or even more complex behaviour involved in aggression, dominance, leadership and social adaptability.

Organismic variables

Are characteristic ways in which the particular groups of organism under observation vary. For example, organisms classified according to color of hair, males or females. Mainly refers to the physical, physiological and psychological characteristics of organisms.

Discrete and continous variables

Values of discrete are always exact for example if we observe and record that a subject make eight correct responses, there is no uncertainty with respect to this value. Values of continous are never exact because no matter how accurately we measure the variable there is always uncertainty with respect to the observed or recorded value of variable.

Qualitative and quantitative variable

All continous and discrete variables are quantitative variables because the differences between the possible values of such variables are matters of degree. These are ordered variables where values of such variables can be ordered on a continuum where the relationships of =, >, < will hold true.

Qualitative or unordered variables are variables in which differences in the possible values are matters of kind rather than degree. For example- colour of hair.

SCHEME OF PSYCHOLOGICAL EXPERIMENT

Every psychological experiment is carried out to test the hypothesis. So role of hypothesis in a psychological experiment is important.

Hypothesis

A hypothesis is defined as a suggested answer to a problem. Hypothesis is a result of creative thinking which develops from trial and error learning proceeds through four stages:

1. *preparation*: when a person observes facts and receives training
2. *incubation*: the conscious or unconscious continuance of associational activities
3. *inspiration*: when the material suddenly seems to organize itself.
4. *verification or revision*: where one evaluates and revises the idea

Hypotheses have their beginnings from facts and theories. There were facts first, from the observation of facts, man began to classify and put together in a systematic manner. As more and more facts were accumulated and classified, the patterns of natural laws began to take shape and at man could predict to some extent the occurrence of nature about him. He began to know that this plus this leads to this. From above discussion we can say that hypothesis come from experience.

Important requirements

The hypothesis should be clear cut in its meaning and must fit the problem so as to provide one answer to the one problem stated. Elements of the hypothesis should be simpler. The hypothesis the simpler is the experiment to test its validity. A hypothesis must be verifiable. A hypothesis should be stated in such a way that it gets proved by an experiment if disproves, it loses its right to called as a good hypothesis.

Every psychological experiment raises a problem. Experiment usually begins when there is a problem. E.g. there are different beliefs about the effects of smoking. Some people believe that it helps in concentrating. Other say that it is not smoking but the personality of a person. This discussion creates a problem about the effect of smoking on physical and mental capacity. Next step is defining and analyzing a problem. One has to define each word of the problem. E.g. what the experiments mean by smoking, mental and physical capacity. Next is to guess the solution of a problem in a statement form. Thus, the hypothesis would be like this—smoking is harmful for mental and physical health. Further, forming an experimental design:

(a) the variables to be studied under what conditions
(b) describing the apparatus
(c) outlining the procedure to be followed in the interpretation of results.

Then there is observation of the facts. One must observe the facts closely, carefully and stepwise. Recording whatever being observed systematically. Last step is interpretation and discussion i.e., making statistical computations and evaluating the results and then discussing them. And presentation of the results through graphs, tables that are used to summarize the basic findings and making conclusions.

Experimental Design

Experimental design is used for verifying equipment, measuring instruments and planning the steps for conducting experiment and collecting data also. In an experiment, meaningful relationships can be established between antecedents and consequences. Among the antecedents are the conditions present in the environment and in the organism called as independent variable.

Independent variable (IV)

- IVs are imposed on the subject at the time of experiment by experimenter.
- IVs are all those aspects of the experiment which the experiment varies systematically.
- IV is marked off in units of intensity, time trials and so forth and scaled accordingly on the baseline of any graph for displaying the results of the experiment.
- IV in one experiment will be merely one of many antecedent conditions which is to be held constant in another experiment.

Dependent variable (DV)

The consequences of the experiment are dependent variable.

- DVs are the measures of the response of the organism whether these may be enumerations of error or correct performance, magnitude, or speed of reaction as contraction of the pupil, electrophysiological changes evolved by the changes in the heart rate.
- DVs are considered to be the main result of the experiment.

Constant variable

Constant variables are those aspects of the experiment that are not under primary study which are inner environment, characteristics of the subject. Example: experimental constants include temperature, conditions of lighting, quietness, special provisions for the experiment such as comfortable seating and adequate communication between subject and experimenter.

Extraneous variables

Extraneous variables, irrelevant variables, secondary variables, nuisance variables etc are all the variables other than the independent variable whose effect is being studied in the experiment. Experimenter tries to control these extraneous variables which may influence the results. They are controlled through randomization, elimination, matching, statistical control methods. Kinds of extraneous variables which are required to be controlled are:

1. Situational variables are the environmental variables operating in the experimental situations. E.g. Light, noise, etc.
2. Subject variable: most variables having to do with the experimental task facing the subject.
3. Sequence relevant variable: arise when the subjects are tested under two or more conditions of the experiment in a sequence which can affect the subject's performances under more than one condition and under the other condition controlled by counterbalancing.

Relevant variables

The previous studies which have determined the relevance of certain variables which must be considered for control in an experiment are called relevant variables.

Intervening variable

Intervening variable is a concept. It is a product of the experimenter's observations and his comparisons of other sets of information. They are hypothetical entities which help the experimenter to think about the relations between antecedents (IV) and consequences (DV). Intervening variables cannot be observed directly. To study the link between IV and DV an indirect approach is to be followed. These are the extractions of larger data of our observations which explain the relation between the IV and DV. They are useful in interpreting the results.

The essential process of conducting the experiment is as follows:

1. Experimenter varies the IV in a systematic manner.
2. He controls the extraneous variables through several methods-randomization, matching, elimination, counterbalancing.
3. Further, he studies previous literature containing observations which are related to his present experiment. And tries to control the relevant variables. Certain other factors or variables are kept constant such characteristics of the subject and inner environment.
4. And, then the effect of the IV is observed on the variable which is DV. These observations are to be recorded systematically. In interpreting the results the intervening variable helps. Intervening variables help the experimenter to think about the relation between IV and DV.

TYPES OF EXPERIMENTAL DESIGN

Single Case Experimental Design

Single case experimental designs are an outgrowth of applied clinical research especially in the area of behaviour modification. In single case experimental design, the objective is to study intensively a particular individual rather than a group of individuals. Repeated measurements are taken across time on one particular individual to note the subtle changes in behaviour.

Advantage

Provide such information about human behaviour that is not always obtainable in group designs. They are useful in clinical research especially in area of behaivour modification.

Disadvantage

Single case experimental designs do not lend themselves to clear statistical analysis. Secondly, hypothesis testing cannot be formalized. The experimenter cannot control the order effects. Lastly, this design does not provide a good basis for generalization.

Quasi Experimental Design

Quasi experimental designs are the plan of such experiments where the experimenter has no control over the selection of subjects and also over the assignment of subjects to the treatments. Further, the experimenter could not manipulate the independent variable as the IV already occurs.

Advantage

It is possible to seek answer to several kinds of problems about past situations and those situations which cannot be handled by employing experimental design.

Disadvantage

Random assignment of subjects to the treatment is not possible and it was therefore a handicap in controlling secondary variables. Such experimental investigations are less powerful in drawing causal relationships between IV and DV.

Experimental Designs

Include all those experiments where:

—large number of experimental units or subjects are to be studied.

—the subjects are randomly assigned to the treatment plan

—independent variable is manipulated by the experimenter and the

—experimenter has full control over the scheduling of independent variables.

This category can be classified into two types of experiments. One in which the investigator manipulates only one variable and studies its effect on another variable DV.

When an experiment focuses only on the influence of a single conditions which can be either present or absent (such a condition) where IV with two values, one representing its presence, the other is its absence. In this case, the simple experimental design calls for an experimental group with the condition present and a control condition with the condition absent. Technique of analysis of variance is used to compare two groups. Second, is multivariate experiment where studies involve simultaneous manipulation of several variables. Technique of analysis of variance is used to study simultaneous influence of more than one variable.

Advantage: They are used when it becomes necessary to study how several I.V. interact to produce an effect one or even on several D.V. Frequently used in psychological research.

Disadvantage: Studies are complicated.

There are three types of experimental designs

1. *Between subjects design*: where each subject is observed only under one of the several treatment conditions.
2. *Within subjects design*: or repeated measures design

   Where each subject is observed under all the treatment conditions involved in the experiment.
3. *Mixed design*: where some factors are b/w subjects and some within subjects are observed.

ADVANTAGES AND LIMITATIONS OF EXPERIMENTAL METHOD

Advantages

1. One major advantage of this method is their replication. If replication is not possible, the experimental findings cannot be confirmed. A dramatic discovery may be reported, but if it cannot be replicated by other scientists it will be rejected.
2. As the experiments can be replicated they become generally acceptable.
3. Replication makes it possible for other experimentalists to draw out more and more findings about the same experiment.
4. Experimental method allows maximum control over the investigation.
5. Since an experiment can be done in a pre-arranged systematic manner, observations can be made in a precise and accurate way.
6. It is possible to isolate a genuine cause for behaviour in a more definite manner.

Limitations

1. It is an artificial situation.
2. The experimental data obtained under artificial set up may not reveal natural and actual working of mental processes under normal condition.
3. Human behaviour is complex and what is observed in an experiment may be inadequate.
4. The motivation to perform well may influence the performance of a task under experimental situation and the result may not be accurate.
5. Behaviour is extremely variable. More over, no two individuals are alike so results or findings cannot be always generalized.
6. A physicist can duplicate the conditions of his experiment like temperature and pressure but psychologist cannot keep the amount of experience same of the subject.
7. Experimenters cannot work with same subject: he comes to know their characteristics and control of their past experiences.
8. Experimental method cannot be used when a researcher wants to study human brain.

APPLICATION OF EXPERIMENTAL METHODS IN OTHER BRANCHES OF PSYCHOLOGY

1. In clinical psychology – it is used in behaviour modification technique.
2. Psychologists administer and interpret intelligence, achievement and conduct personality tests. Moreover help teachers to change their methods of training.
3. Psychologists conduct experiments: They design machines so that human errors can be minimized. Psychologists conduct experiments to judge whether the accused is mentally competent to stand trial.
4. Psychologists plan the design and analyze data of large scale experiments & surveys.

REFLECT YOURSELF

1. What are the different applications of experimental method?
2. Discuss the various types of variables.
3. List various advantages and disadvantages of experimental method.
4. What is the variable?
5. What is an experiment?
6. Give an example of intervening variable.

21

PSYCHOLOGICAL TESTING

TOPICS COVERED IN THIS CHAPTER

- Introduction
- Characteristics of a Psychological Test
- Uses of Psychological Testing
- Standards for Testing

INTRODUCTION

The roots of psychological testing can be traced back to ancient times. Over 3,000 years ago Chinese used written tests in filling "civil service" posts. At the turn of the eighteenth century towards nineteenth century contributions by following pioneers are: Francis Galton stimulated investigations of individual differences and also directed his experimental efforts to measure intelligence by means of tests of imagery and sensory discriminations. He advised a test for the measurement of the delicacy of weight discrimination. In 1905 Binet devised a test to measure differences in mental development-in degree of brightness or dullness with differences in the level of development. He gave impetus to the study of individual differences by means of standardized tests. James Mc Keen Cattell much younger than Galton but still his contemporary. It was Cattell who first employed the term "mental tests". Cattell's tests were of memory, imagery, keenness of eye sight, colour preferences and reaction time. The great development in testing and studying individual differences in the United States occurred after Binet's work was made known. Goddard was the first to revise Binet scales: Later Terman who also contributed in revising. Binet scale and presented the scale in its standardized directions for administering and scoring.

Psychological test represent the test, fairest and accurate technology available for making decisions about individuals. "Psychological test is a measurement instrument that has three defining characterists:

1. A psychological test is a sample of behaviour.
2. The sample obtained under standardized condition.

3. There are established rules for scoring for obtaining quantitative information from the behaviour sample, according to Murphy and Shofer.

"A psychological test is a standardized instrument designed to measure objectively one or more aspects of a total personality by means of sample of verbal or non-verbal responses or by means of other behaviour," as proposed by Freeman.

According to Anastasi, "a psychological test is essentially an objective and standardized measure of a sample of behaviour".

CHARACTERISTICS OF A PSYCHOLOGICAL TEST

(*a*) A psychological test is a sample of behaviour. *i.e.*, A psychological test attempts to approximate the exhaustive procedure of measuring all possible behaviour used in measuring a particular attribute by collecting a systematic sample of behaviour.

Secondly such behaviour samples measure psychological variables such that the quality of a test is largely determined by the representativeness of this sample. For example: To develop a test of writing ability would not mean to collect and evaluate everything that a person has written from term papers to laundry lists. This is impractical and also it does not the qualify for a test. To ensure practicality and representativeness of the behaviour includes a series of short essays, sample letters, memos etc., which makes more meaningful.

(*b*) The sample is obtained under standardized conditions also scored and interpreted under standardized procedures. Standardized administration includes the following example: The scholastic aptitude test is administered to thousands of students. Here, a test supervisor reads detailed instructions to all examinees before starting and each portion of test is timed. Test manual includes exhaustive instruction dealing with appropriate seating patterns, lighting, interruptions and emergencies, standardized scoring procedure: Includes same set of scoring rules applied to many people taking the same test. Standardized interpretation of test score: includes the way test scores are interpreted. The role of the examiner should be minimized.

(*c*) Psychological tests are designed to measure specific attributes of persons not the whole person.

(*d*) They only tell us ways in which individuals are similar or different.

(*e*) Psychological tests are invariably imperfect. *i.e.*, they may not provide an adequate measure of a specific attribute, of two people. For example, John may receive a high score than Mary on a test of spatial ability. In fact, he may have equal ability as that of Mary.

(*f*) Psychological tests are reliable to an extent. *i.e.*, they do provide an adequate measure of a particular attribute assigns nears in a consistent fashion. There are methods which determine reliability.

These are:

1. **Test retest method:** It is the oldest. It involves administering a test to a group of individuals and read ministering same test to the same group at later time. Then correlating first set of scores with the second. If correlation is high, then the test is said to be reliable.

2. **Alternate Forms method:** It involves administering one form of the test to a group of individuals at some later time administering an alternate form of the same test, to the same group. Then correlating scores of 2 forms.
3. **Split-Half method:** This method involves administering a test to a group of individuals splitting the test in half and then correlating scores on one half of even items with scores on other half of odd items.
4. **Internal consistency method:** It involves administering a test to a group of individuals and completing correlations among all items and computing average of intercorrelations.

(*g*) Tests are used to make inferences about people. There are two types of inferences which one might make on the basis of test scores. First, there are inferences regarding the attribute being measured. Secondly, inference regarding the decisions about individuals. These inferences are called validity of measurement and validity of decisions respectively.

(*h*) Psychological tests are scored on basis of standardized norms, according to which test scores become significant. A norm based score indicates where an individual stands in comparison to the particular normative group that defines the set of standards. The norms are empirically established by determining what a representative group of persons actually do on the test.

There are different types of norms:

1. ***Age-norms*:** An age norm relates a level of test performance to the age of people who have taken the test. Many psychological characteristics change over time like vocabulary, mathematical ability etc.

   Advantages:

   - Applicable for any trait (psychological or physical) which changes with age upto some age level, easy to use, familiar term, Convenient to use and easy to understand.

   Limitations:

   - Psychological characteristics which don't change with age can't have Age norms. The rate of growth and age of reaching the maximum growth is different for different abilities; we cannot compare different growth curves. Age norms have inequality of units of measurements. There is inequality in growth rate as rate of development is different at every age.

2. ***Grade norms*:** It is a type of norm commonly used in school settings. Grade norms are found by computing the mean raw score obtained by children in each grade. Hence, the reference point is the class in which he/she studies unlike age norms where chronological age forms the baseline of the graph. They tells us how much the person has learnt knowledge in a certain field?

   Applied only to subjects which are taught in the subjects school or college.

   Advantages: technical in application, convenient in usage and familiar with people.

   Limitations: Grade norms cannot be regarded as performance standards.

   They are not comparable between different schools, between students of different grade. There is inequality of measurement. Even within the same grade, norms set separately for 2 different abilities cannot be compared. For eg.: reading is different from writing-grade norms for a grade depends upon course being taught, method of teaching and students ability.

3. *Percentile norms*: They designate percentage of cases lying below a certain raw score. A percentile indicates the individual's relative position in the standardization sample. Percentiles can also be regarded as ranks in a group of 10, except that in ranking it is customary to start counting at the top, the best person in the group receiving a rank of one. With percentiles, we count from the bottom, the lower the percentile, the poorer the individuals standing.

   Advantages: They provide convenient land marks for describing a distribution of scores and comparing it with other distribution. Useful for a layman also. Easy to compute.

   Limitations -inequality in their units, especially at the extremes of the distribution. Discrepancy in the gaps between percentiles ranks are, inequal.–If the reference group is changed, the percentile rank gets changed.

4. *Standard scores*: Standard scores express the individuals distance from the mean in terms of the standard deviation of the distribution. They can be obtained by either linear or non-linear transformation of the raw scores. When obtained by linear transformations, then retain the exact numerical relations of the original raw scores because they are computed by subtracting a constant from each raw score and then dividing the result by another constant.

   Zscore = X-X

   X-mean.-S.D. of the normative group, X-individuals raw score

Profiles: are graphical representation of a set of scores for the same individual expressed in same units of measurement. The main purpose of the profile is to allow the examinee to compare his or her profile with patterns that are typical for individuals who are considered successful in different occupations. Note: Psychological test norms are in no sense absolute, universal or permanent. They merely represent the test performance of the persons constituting the standardized sample.

USES OF PSYCHOLOGICAL TESTING

Educational Testing

Admissions and advancement of students in schools and institutions.

- Placement of variety of special education program.
- Diagnosing learning difficulties in children
- Assessment and evaluation of the effectiveness of different curricula.
- Publication of avg. test results for each school to account for a drive in education
- Test results can be used in allocating funds to different schools for a remedial education.
- Certifying graduates.

Personal Testing

Ability tests and tests of specific skills are used. Ability tests are used for screening new volunteers and for optimum placement of solutions according to their skills or abilities:

- Tests are used to assess training needs, individual
- Workers performance in training,

- Success of training programs.
- Tests can be used as part of a management development and career counseling program.

Clinical Testing

Clinical psychologists employ neuropsychological test-batteries.

- Tests are also used in diagnosing many types of brain damage.
- Discover personal problems in learning. Etc.

STANDARDS FOR TESTING

The American Psychological Association (APA) has taken a leading role in developing professional standards for testing. There are documents which deal with several issues. These are -The ethical principles of psychologists: it outlines the psychologist's responsibility with regard to competence, confidentiality and welfare of consumers of psychological services.

- Standards for educational and psychological testing-outlines the technical and professional standards to be followed in construction, evaluation, interpretation, and application.
- Principles for the validation and use of personnel selection procedures. speciality guidelines -outlines professional standards for clinical, counseling, industrial organizational and school psychologists.

REFLECT YOURSELF

1. What the different uses of psychological tests?
2. Delineate the characteristics of psychological tests.

22

INTERVIEW METHOD

TOPICS COVERED IN THIS CHAPTER
• Introduction • Interview and Interview Schedule are Classified • Criteria for Question Writing

INTRODUCTION

Interview schedule is a tool of social sciences. It involves a set of questions related to social, political and cognitive issues. It is a tool to get information from the respondent concerning various psychological and sociological issues. Interview means, "conversation with a purpose" by Bingham and Moore, 1941.

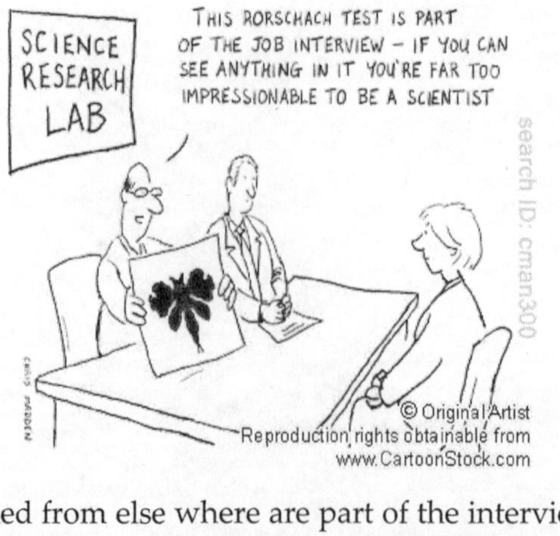
SCIENCE RESEARCH LAB
THIS RORSCHACH TEST IS PART OF THE JOB INTERVIEW – IF YOU CAN SEE ANYTHING IN IT YOU'RE FAR TOO IMPRESSIONABLE TO BE A SCIENTIST
search ID: cman300
© Original Artist
Reproduction rights obtainable from
www.CartoonStock.com

Data which could be attained from else where are part of the interview record (e.g. test scores, bio-graphical information, letters of recommendation) make this process on the upper edge of other selection devices. Secondly, data which are unique to the interview process are (personal dress and general mannerism).

There are many studies which reflect the importance of interview. One of them is quoted below:

Spriegel & James (1958) examined the data from both a 1930 survey of 236 firms and 1957 survey of 852 firms in the earlier survey, 93% of the firms reported using an interview as part of their selection process; by 1957 it increased to 99%.

Interviews used in industry differ according to their objectives. Some of the different objectives are:

- It may be used as an exploratory device to identify variables and study hypothesis.
- It is used as a supplementary device to validate other methods. E.g. questionnaire method.
- It is used as a main instrument for studying relationship among various variables and hypothesis.
- To evaluate the candidate for purposes of hiring, promotion or transfer. Such interviews are referred to as selection or placement interviews.
- To obtain information concerning the employee's attitude about his/her job, the company etc. These interviews are referred to as attitude interviews.
- Many interviews are carried out during employment or at the point of termination. Such interviews are called as exit or separation interviews.
- To provide help on-the-job, such interviews are called as counseling interviews.
- To evaluate the employee under difficult situation. Such interviews are called as assessment or stress interviews.

Despite these objectives, interview often is difficult to evaluate as a selection device because the purpose of the interviews is:

- To gather as much data relevant to the selection.
- To evaluate the data available and decide whether to select or reject the applicant.
- Type of interviews
- Degree of training which the interviewer has received
- His biases
- The position he is directed to fill
- Duration of the interview
- Behaviour of the interview should be standardized from applicant to applicant.
- Symonds (1939) has listed a series of factors which he believes can influence the quality and quantity of data collected during interview.
    1. Factors inherent in the applicant: age, intelligence, sex, race, socioeconomic level, language ability, emotional quotient, security, applicants attitude toward interviewer, applicant's previous acquaintance with interviews and purpose of applicant in coming to the interview.
    2. Factors inherent in the interviewer: age, sex, intelligence, race, socioeconomic level, position with reference to the applicant, personality (sociability, sympathy, empathy, human interest and credibility), social outlook, psychological understanding (ability to sense or feel the purposes, needs or drives of the applicant), previous acquaintance,

interest of interviewer to applicant (degree to which interviewer enjoys the conversation of interviewer).

3. Situational factors such as: place, time, person's present, first, second or subsequent interview experience of applicant directly preceeding interview, emergency character of interview, directions given applicant preceeding the interview and voluntary versus non-voluntary nature of interview.
4. Factors in the form and content of interview: content of questions, form of questions, interpretation, suggestion or other reactions of interviewer, purpose of the interview, identity of the interviewer, encouragement given by the interviewer, remarks interpolated by examiner during the interview.

INTERVIEW AND INTERVIEW SCHEDULE ARE CLASSIFIED

(*a*) **Structured interview:** List of questions to be asked (are prepared already) in the same order. Structured interviews are also referred to as patterned interviews.

(*b*) **Unstructured interview:** Where list of questions may be there, but not asked sequentially. The interviewer is free to ask in any order.

In both these types interviews schedule has 3 kinds of information:

1. Identification data: face, name, status, region and political
2. Sociological variables: income, status, region and political affiliation, occupation level, education level.
3. Problem information: information concerning the main problem which is to be studied.

The types of items which are used in order to get information on sociological and psychological variables are of three kinds. These are:

- fixed alternative
- open-end question
- scale item

Fixed alternative: Questions are framed in such a way that the options in which the respondent has to answer is fixed.

Advantage: Information can be easily coded. There is uniformity of measurement i.e. everybody responds in the same order and same category.

Limitations: Information obtained may be very superficial. Respondent may get irritated because they are interested in giving more information than responding into yes or no. further, individuals may not respond in a sincere manner.

Open-end questions: Where respondent is free to give any answer in 3 or 4 statements or a paragraph.

Advantage: The interviewer gets information pertaining to personal issues. It is quite flexible i.e. questions can be adjusted according to the respondent and study of subject. The interviewer puts a minimum restrain on the respondent in answering because there are no fixed categories. There is possibility of depth in answers and the investigator can study the issue in detail. Further, while probing one can clear up the misunderstanding. The interviewer can detect respondent's lack of knowledge. These type of questions can be used to detect ambiguity. It also encourages cooperation. One can study hypothesis which can be later on studied.

Limitation: It is time consuming. As the job of interviewer is to first code the information and then tabulate. It is not economical. It is expensive as lot of energy and time is invested in it. Further, there is no uniformity of responses.

Scale item: Scaling of answering is somewhat like this: agree, somewhat agree, seldom agree and never agree. Such a scaling procedure is used mostly in attitude scale.

Advantage: There is uniformity of responses. The only differences are that there are more categories. Information can be easily coded.

Limitation: Too much analytic approach is required.

CRITERIA FOR QUESTION WRITING

- Is the question related to the research problem?
- Is the type of question right? That is, whether scale, open-ended will be suitable. It depends upon the issue studied.
- Is the language unambiguous i.e. is it precise and clear?
- Is the question leading? In leading questions where the respondent gives obvious answer, such as do you read newspaper? Such questions should be avoided.
- Does the question demands knowledge. Such questions should also avoided because sometimes the respondent lack certain level of knowledge. In such cases, first give a para to assess whether the person has certain level of information.
- Does the question demand personal information regarding open issue such as marriage. Such questions should be avoided.
- Is the question loaded with social desirability? Such questions should be avoided for e.g. do you like to help?

  Question writing is a skill and demand experience.

Evaluation of Interview and Interview Schedule

In terms of reliability and validity, we have to consider a lot many factors. These are: training of interviewers, type of question written (should be precise and simple), lack of sharp and constant focus on problem and hypothesis, lack of appreciation of schedule as a measurement instrument, lack of necessary background and experience. It should be objective about how attitude change and develops, knowledge about persuasion and sensitive towards issues. Further, it has great potential in yielding data. Any kind of problem can be studied through interview method. Body language, facial expressions and way of responding can be noted. It is adaptable. It is suitable to all kinds of respondents. One limitation it has is that it is expensive. Despite its limitation, both as a selection technique and a tool for research purposes. It is suitable to any kind of issue and respondent. Interview can be a group or individual interviews. As both interviewer could examine each candidate together working as a team. Each interviewer could examine each candidate separately and then hire or reject after the agreement of other interviewer.

Dont's of the interview process

Failure to establish rapport with the candidate: Rapport does not mean making friends with the candidate. Neither is it about playing psychologist to the candidate's anxieties.

Not knowing exactly what abilities are required; not working from a meticulously developed list of requirement. Relying upon job descriptions will not be a sufficient way when the interviewer also needs to know what abilities and soft skills are required for a particular job and specific position which the candidate may hold in the hierarchy of organization.

Becoming a victim of the halo effect; halo effect may arise when the interviewer finds something in common with the interviewee such as hailing from same college, state or even religion.

Doing most of the talking; if the interviewer fails to listen then he/she is missing the entirely important and meaningful information from the candidate. This can happen when the interviewer talks too much and listen less.

Not allowing silences to occur. The only way the interviewer can influence a reluctant candidate to speak is by keeping silent with body language.

Asking questions that serve no purpose: it means that if the interviewer asks irrelevant questions just to fill up the time. And this gives a hint to the candidate to recognize that the interviewer is engaged in question generation rather than listening to them.

Poor sequencing of questions: if the interview is not planned then the interviewer will jump around from one domain to other domain.

Making impulsive conclusions and generalizations based on some assumed characteristic. It may happen when the interviewer base his judgment on the physical appearance, diction and values.

Repeating the information on the application or resume; it wastes a lot of time but it is an excellent way to interview the candidate when one is not prepared to do so.

Ignoring intuition (gut-feeling)

These are the feelings which result from facts, observation (candidate's body language) and experience coming together on a subconscious level. Intuition is a sign which needs more definitive information.

Asking questions that don't give worthwhile information; this category includes (1) questions that telegraph the desired responses (listening skills), (2) apparent choices where there are none i.e. do you get emotional and overreact or can you keep a cool head and questions where the answers, although obvious cannot be checked for truthfulness.

Asking "magic question"; these questions are penetrative in nature about the candidate's personality e.g. if you could be an animal, which one would you choose?

Not being knowledgeable about the legal restrictions regarding interviewing; it includes the desired level of knowledge about legal matter. If the interviewer is unclear about what can and cannot be asked he or she may fail to do a thorough interview out of fear of delving into an illegal topic.

Giving evaluative feedback; exchanging opinion with the candidate. The interview situation is not a social event as his/her opinions are not a concern here.

Asking multiple choice (laundry list) questions; such pattern of questions will give the opportunity to the candidate to escape the task of thinking by simply selecting a response from the list of choices provided by the interviewer.

Excessive note taking; taking notes in bulk will confuse the interviewer. Moreover, he/she will fail to take notice of candidate's body language, facial expressions, tone and other miscellaneous gestures.

Giving commitments; making promises. For example, unintentional comments such as "I think you will be hired" will be treated as hiring commitments. And if the candidate not hired, then candidate may claim that he/she was guaranteed employment.

REFLECT YOURSELF

1. Define interview method?
2. What is an interview schedule?
3. What are the different types of response sets?
4. What are the different types of interview?
5. Question writing is a skill. Discuss.

23

CASE STUDY

TOPICS COVERED IN THIS CHAPTER
• Introduction • Types of Case Studies • Sources of Information Used in a Case Study

INTRODUCTION

A case study is an in-depth study of one person. The other form of research that psychologists frequently use in their work is called a case study. Unlike a survey, a case study closely studies one individual as opposed to a group of individuals. Case studies can be compared and contrasted to help further analyze data. Case studies were developed from the idea of single cases being tried in a court of law. Sigmund Freud was the first in his field to use case studies to learn more about his patients. Individual case studies helped Sigmund Freud to develop most of his work and theories.

The benefits of performing a case study include getting an in-depth view into a subject's behaviour and can also help a psychologist determine research questions to study for larger group. A disadvantage to doing a case study is that a psychologist may start off only looking for certain data and accidentally overlook important behaviours while only focusing on desired data, or data may be purposely overlooked if it does not coincide with an original hypothesis. Finding willing participants can sometimes prove difficult. Case studies are generally a single-case design, but can also be a multiple-case design, where replication instead of sampling is the criterion for inclusion. Like other research methodologies within psychology, the case study must produce valid and reliable results in order to be useful for the development of future research. Further, with the case study it is impossible to generalize the findings to a wider population of people. The hope is that learning gained from studying one case can be generalized to many others. Unfortunately, case studies tend to be highly subjective and it is harder to generalize results to a larger population. The case study method cannot set precedent for all cases with like patients. For example, a case study on patient John Smith, a psychopath, cannot necessarily create a universal principal that applies to all other psychopaths. This is one of the downsides that the case study method presents.

In a case study, nearly every aspect of the subject's life and history is analyzed to seek patterns and causes for behaviour. A case study is study conducted using an individual client or patient who is undergoing treatment (Trull, 2005). This method of psychological research has long been regarded as one of clinician's most valuable resources in gaining understanding of a patient's condition. Cases as "The Case of Dora (Freud, 1905)," "The Case of Little Hans (Freud, 1909)," "The Three Faces of Eve (Thigpen and Cleckley, 1957)," "The Mask of Sanity (Cleckley, 1964)", and "Cases in Behaviour Modification (Ullman and Krasner, 1965)" have all given clinicians a critical and crucial look into the behaviours and lives of different abnormal minds.

It is important to understand that no one research method can definitely examine a psychological illness. However, case studies over history of psychology have been able to provide clinicians with valuable information about different psychological illnesses. Meaning, a particular study can be used as a means of insight into life with the illness, thoughts of the patient; and the formation of hypothesis on behaviour, treatments, and further research on the issue at hand. This information is gathered through interviews, test responses, diaries, medical history, biographical and autobiographical accounts and data, treatment responses, etc. (Trull, 2005).

Another downside to the case study method is the completely open and uncontrolled environment in which it takes place. This eliminates it's usefulness as an indicator of cause and effect since the variables in the study are uncontrolled. This makes it too difficult to state that one value correlates in any way to another. Instead, a clinician can develop a hypothesis on this relationship and use another research method to determine support for, or refutation for, their hypothesis. This is why it was mentioned earlier that case studies can lay down the foundations for further psychological research.

Today, case studies are still highly valued. Former case studies drive psychological education, and current studies expand our understanding of the patient and condition, while opening up new avenues of research. A case study is a very intimate and critical means of understanding an individual patient, especially a severely complex one. Thus, despite the limitations of case studies, they stand as an extremely useful method of psychological research.

TYPES OF CASE STUDIES

- Explanatory: Such case studies used to do causal investigations.
- Exploratory: A case study that is sometimes used as a prelude to further, more in-depth research. This allows researchers to gather more information before developing their research questions and hypotheses.
- Descriptive: Involves starting with a descriptive theory. The subjects are then observed and the information gathered is compared to the pre-existing theory.
- Intrinsic: A type of case study in which the researcher has a personal interest in the case.
- Collective: Involves studying a group of individuals.
- Instrumental: Occurs when the individual or group allows researchers to understand more than what is initially obvious to observers.

Case Study Methods

- Prospective: A type of case study in which an individual or group of people is observed in order to determine outcomes. For example, a group of individuals might be watched over an extended period of time to observe the progression of a particular disease.
- Retrospective: A type of case study that involves looking at historical information. For example, researchers might start with an outcome, such as a disease, and then backwards at information about the individual's life to determine risk factors that may have contributed to the onset of the illness.

SOURCES OF INFORMATION USED IN A CASE STUDY

There are a number of different sources and methods that researchers can use to gather information about an individual or group. The six major sources that have been identified by researchers (Yin, 1994; Stake, 1995) are:

- Direct observation: This strategy involves observing the subject, often in a natural setting. While an individual observer is sometimes used, it is more common to utilize a group of observers.
- Interviews: One of the most important methods for gathering information in case studies. An interview can involve structured survey-type questions, or more open-ended questions.
- Documents: Letters, newspaper articles, administrative records, etc.
- Archival records: Census records, survey records, name lists, etc.
- Physical artifacts: Tools, objects, instruments and other artifacts often observed during a direct observation of the subject.
- Participant observation: Involves the researcher actually serving as a participant in events and observing the actions and outcomes.

Case Study, at a glance	
Advantages	**Disadvantages**
• Detailed in-depth information concerning a person, a family, an organization or an event. • High ecological validity. • Sensitive to the individual, and sensitive issues concerning the individual.	• Cannot generalise results. • Replication impossible, to confirm earlier results. • Reliability of information obtained by self-report. • Interviewer/observer bias. • Lack of scientific validity. • No cause-effect conclusions can be made.

REFLECT YOURSELF

1. Define case study.
2. From which school of thought does case study approach got its impetus?
3. What are the different types of case studies?
4. Define prospective and retrospective research.
5. Name few famous cases.
6. List the advantages and drawbacks using a case study method.

24

FIELD OBSERVATION

TOPICS COVERED IN THIS CHAPTER

- Introduction
- Guide to Doing Field Observation

INTRODUCTION

We watch other people in the environment but we don't do it in order to derive information about their people behaviour. This is what social sciences look at. Observation involves looking and listening to what other people say or behave.

What is Field Observation?

There are many types of observation methods. But here field observation is discussed in detail. Participant observation is a qualitative method with roots in traditional ethnographic research. Participant observation or field observation is one of the most demanding and common methods of qualitative data collection method. It requires the researcher to become a participant in the specific culture or context under study. Participant observation often requires months or years of intensive work because the researcher needs to become accepted as a natural part of the culture in order to assure that the observations are part of natural phenomenon.

Field observation is different from laboratory observation or non-participant observation in a number of ways. First, the non participant observer doesn't typically try to become a participant in the culture under study. The researcher is watching rather than taking part. Technology can be a useful part of direct observation or non participant observation. For instance, one can videotape the phenomenon or observer from behind. Here the observer is not bias about his observations. Third, is non-participant observer tends to be more focused than participant observation. Here, the researcher manipulates the independent variable under study. The field observer takes his observations in a natural setting. Non-participant observer is taking the observation in an artificial setting. Another disadvantage of participant observation is the difficulty of documenting the data – it is hard to write down everything that is important while you are in the act of participating and observing. The non-participant observation tends not to take as long as participant observation. It is so because the laboratory conditions are set where the independent variable is manipulated by the experimenter. So cannot be continued to for long as experimental conditions are not met for such durations. Finally, in field observation it requires conscious effort at objectivity because method is inherently subjective.

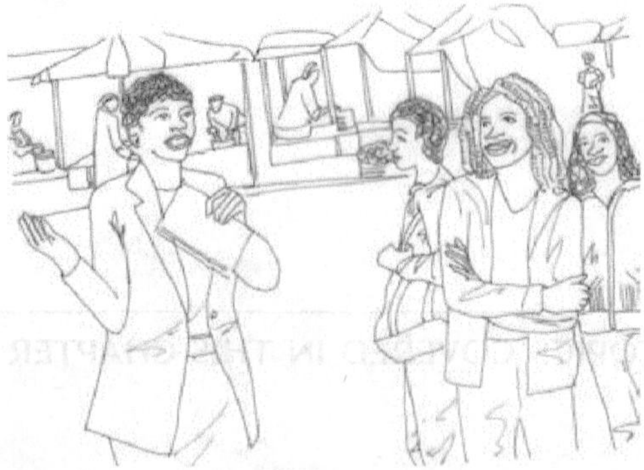

Why use Field Observation Over other Research Methods?

Observation allows the researcher to study people in their natural setting without their behaviour being influenced by the presence of a researcher in a laboratory setting. Field observational data usually consists of detailed information about particular groups or situations. This kind of data can fill out and provide deeper, richer, understanding than a survey work which tends to be less comprehensive about a larger number of people. As in field observation an observer can observe about what a lot of what people do they do it naturally, they aren't aware of it. Other methods of observation allows for the study of one individual at a time. Observation, particularly the field observation enables the research to study groups of people together, *i.e.*, it allows for the study of interactions among people. An interview for instance only shows a person's views at one time. observations involves the study of groups or situations over time, thus revealing changes. For example, school truants may not agree to cooperate with methods of research such as non participant observation or interviews. Sometimes participant observation is the only way of finding out about such groups. Further, it allows for insight into contexts, relationships, behavior and can provide information previously unknown to researchers that is crucial for project design, data-collection, and interpretation of other data. Researchers use data collected through participant observation to improve the design of other methods, such as interviews and focus groups. For instance, they help to ensure the cultural relevance and appropriateness of interview and focus group questions.

How can Participant Observation be Used?

Following questions will be used for field observation:

- What groups or situations would be relevant?
- Is it possible and practical to observe them?

- Should you use non-participant or participant observation?
- What could you find out from the observation?
- If you are doing field observation you will have to decide whether to remain hidden – not tell anyone that you are observing them and be open–tell people that you are observing them.

GUIDE TO DOING FIELD OBSERVATION

- Make arrangements necessary for the observation to take place. Where you should go to do participant observation depends on the research goals. Generally, you should try to go where people in the study population often go in their daily lives, and engage in the activity of interest. A key informant could tell you where those places are. For example, you might go where people in the study population seek medical care, socialize, eat, or shop. You could visit places where high-risk sexual activities are negotiated, such as discotheques or bars. Another option is to attend organized events such as religious services, municipal activities, and public information sessions.
- Ask for permission well in advance if you want to arrange a visit. At the beginning stages of a research project, participant observation is used to facilitate and develop positive relationships among researchers and key informants, stakeholders, and gate keepers, whose assistance and approval are needed for the study to become a reality. These relationships are essential to the logistics of setting up the study, including gaining permission from appropriate officials, and identifying and gaining access to potential study participants.
- Plan the days in advance and the duration for which you will be part of the group.
- Make necessary work sheets with headings that you will use for your notes on observation. Decide exactly what you are trying to find out and work out suitable headings to make notes. Once you have a clear idea of what the research is about, you can determine specific objectives for the participant observation activity. It may be useful to create a list of things to pay attention to, and either write it in your field notebook or keep it in your pocket for quick reference.
- Whom to recruit for the study and how best to recruit them? This question is best answered by field observers. Participant observation may be done individually, in pairs, and in teams – whichever arrangement is most appropriate for covering the locations and topics at issue. Factors often considered in determining the appropriate arrangement include the age, gender, physical appearance, ethnicity, personality, and linguistic abilities of different data collectors. The objective should be to gather data in the least obtrusive and most efficient manner possible, in light of the specific population and context. One way to do participant observation is for members of a team to disperse to different locations individually, or in pairs or groups, to spend time doing focused observation to address particular questions. They can then reconvene to compare notes. From these notes, they can construct a more complete picture of the issues being studied. They might then create a map indicating places where some activity of interest was observed or where certain types of people go at different times of the day or week.

What to Observe During Participant Observation?

Category	Includes	Researchers should note
Appearance	Clothing, age, gender, physical appearance	Anything that might indicate membership in groups or in sub-populations of interest to the study, such as profession, social status, socioeconomic class, religion, or ethnicity
Verbal behaviour and interactions	Who speaks to whom and for how long; who initiates interaction; languages or dialects spoken; tone of voice	Gender, age, ethnicity, and profession of speakers; dynamics of interaction
Physical behaviour and gestures	What people do, who does what, who interacts with whom, who is not interacting	How people use their bodies and voices to communicate different emotions; what individuals' behaviors indicate about their feelings toward one another, their social rank, or their profession
Personal space	How close people stand to one another	What individuals' preferences concerning personal space suggest about their relationships
Human traffic	People who enter, leave, and spend time at the observation site	Where people enter and exit; how long they stay; who they are (ethnicity, age, gender); whether they are alone or accompanied; number of people
People who stand out	Identification of people who receive a lot of attention from others	The characteristics of these individuals; what differentiates them from others; whether people consult them or they approach other people; whether they seem to be strangers or well known by others present.

What form do participants observation data take?

In large part, participant observation data consist of the detailed field notes that the researcher records in a field notebook. Although typically textual, such data may also include maps and other diagrams, such as kinship or organizational charts. Occasionally, participant observation may involve quantification of something and, as a result, produce numerical data. For example, the researcher could count the number of people who enter a particular space and engage in a particular activity during a specified segment of time. Textual notes are entered into computer files, and data of all forms are analyzed and consulted on a regular basis throughout the study, as discussed elsewhere in this module.

How to be an effective participant observer?

- Try not to stand out or to affect the natural flow of activity. One way to do this is to behave in a way similar to the people around you, such as praying in a religious setting or drinking in a bar.
- Simply put, document what you observe, taking care to distinguish it from both your expectations and your interpretation of what you observe. avoid reporting your interpretation rather than an objective account of what you observe. To interpret is to impose your own judgment on what you see. For example, an interpretive description of a street corner might be that it was "dirty and overly crowded." An objective description would be that "there was garbage everywhere and there were so many people around that it was difficult to move." The danger of not separating interpretation from observation is that your interpretations can turn out to be wrong. This can lead to invalid study results.
- Handwritten notes, later converted into computer files, are often the only way to document certain participant observation activities, such as informal or spontaneous interviews, observation, and generally moving about in the field. Notes from participant observation – like those from interviews and focus groups are called "field notes," and they are written directly into field notebooks.

Tips for Taking field notes

Begin each notebook entry with the date, time, place, and type of data collection event.

Leave space on the page for expanding your notes, or plan to expand them on a separate page.

Take notes strategically. It is usually practical to make only brief notes during data collection.Direct quotes can be especially hard to write down accurately. Rather than try to document every detail or quote, write down key words and phrases that will trigger your memory when you expand notes.

Use shorthand. Because you will expand and type your notes soon after you write them, it does not matter if you are the only person who can understand your shorthand system.Use abbreviations and acronyms to quickly note what is happening and being said.

Cover a range of observations. In addition to documenting events and informal conversations, note people's body language, moods, or attitudes; the general environment; interactions among participants; ambiance; and other information that could be relevant.

Sample Field Notes

Site: Capital City Hospital

Data collector: Tommy lee

Typist: George L.

Date: 22-6-04

Start: 07:30 a.m.

End: 10:15 a.m.

When we arrived,we went first to the antenatal clinic where several xxxxxxx projects are located, including xxxx, xxx, and the xxxxxxxx study.The projects occupy rooms on three sides of the large waiting area, which was largely empty.When we arrived there were seven women in the main waiting area, listening to a nurse give a health talk. A few more women arrived as the talk progressed. We were met by Mrs. xxxxxxx, the head nurse, and introduced to several of the other study nurses. There is a small waiting area off the main waiting area for the xxx project, which includes a recently acquired TV/VCR.This was playing when we arrived, and there were a number of women gathered around watching throughout our visit.They have two HIV videos which the staff said are very popular and that the women will stay after their study visits to watch. Monday and Friday are general antenatal clinic days at the hospital and are therefore busier.Tuesday morning is for high-risk clients and the afternoon is a teen pregnancy clinic.On Wednesday clients return for test results. It was unclear to me what happens on Thursday.

Women are tested for STIs, and treatment is provided to both women and their partners; however, men are usually shy about coming to the clinic because it is all women.The nurses prefer to have the partners come to XXX so they can make sure they are treated.The STI clinic has a long wait and is crowded . . .

REFLECT YOURSELF

1. How does observation method different from observation?
2. What is the difference between participant observation and non-participant observation?
3. Which observation type is a part of ethnographic research?
4. What points of consideration are taken into account for taking field notes?
5. What tips will you suggest to a field observer?

25

RATING SCALE

TOPICS COVERED IN THIS CHAPTER
• Introduction • Shortcomings of Rating Scales • Merits of Rating Scale

INTRODUCTION

Rating scales are used in observational studies to assess the quality of some experience or activity. Regardless, of their objective, these scales are frequently used in either of two ways:

(*a*) To record behaviour at frequent intervals throughout a sample of social interaction or

(*b*) To rate the nature of the entire social events after it has completed. They are found in one or a combination of basic forms: the numerical, forced-choice and the graphic rating scale.

Rating scales are used quite frequently in survey research and there are many different kinds of rating scales.

Numerical Rating Scale

Numerical rating scales are employed by behaviour science researchers to record quantified observations of behaviour of individuals, the activities of an entire group, the change in the situation surrounding them and allied data. Although these scales are less reliable and provide more superficial information than category systems, they are sometimes relied upon for practical considerations. Numerical scales involve a series of points which depict varying extents of the dimensions being observed. Fouriezos et al cited a study, in which a rating scale is used to rate the amount of self-oriented need behaviour in the discussion group. Self-oriented need is conceptualized as primarily directed towards the satisfaction of the need itself, irrespective of the effect on the attainment of group goal. The scale has eleven points ranging from 0 (no expression of self-oriented need) to 10 (all behaviour of the self-oriented need type). The ratings describe the extent of self-oriented behaviour each group member revealed during the meeting. Similar end of meeting ratings can also be made on the basis of reflection and recall by the observer. The numerical scales are simple to construct, easy in use and convenient in data analysis. However, they are more susceptible to varied biases and errors than other types of rating scales.

The Forced Choice Scale

The forced choice scale may be in varied forms. Usually, it presents two equally favourable statements about the observed. The observer is required to choose only one of the two statements to describe him. Thus, he may be forced to indicate whether the individual has more of one quality than another of the given pair. "he is energetic" and "he is intelligent". Although this method can overcome the "halo effect", it is time consuming and sometimes resisted by the observer. A forced-choice rating scale will bias results by eliminating the undecideds and/or those with no opinion. Some researchers will purposely leave out the response choice of "undecided," "no opinion," "uncertain," or "don't know." This approach may be reasonable when the researcher has good reason to believe that virtually all subjects have an opinion and you do not want them to "cop out" by indicating they are uncertain.

The Graphic Rating Scale

The graphic rating scale is in the form of a straight line representing a thermometer and presented either horizontally or vertically. The observer is required to make a judgement which frequently reflects either positively or negatively on the observed. An example is as follows. This is a scale which people use to indicate ratings of a particular attribute.

Unpleasant ————————————————————————— pleasant

Shy ————————————————————————————— outgoing

SHORTCOMINGS OF RATING SCALES

Rating scales are susceptible to at least four types of pitfalls: halo effect, error of liniency, error of central tendency and a logical error in rating. Halo effect refers to tendency on the part of the observer to rate the observed on several qualities according to the general impression (or general mental attitude) he has about him. For example, if a person appears to be sociable, he may rated as intelligent. The error of leniency is the tendency on the part of an observer to overestimate (or underestimate) the desirable qualities of the observed when he likes (or dislikes)him for certain reasons. The error of central tendency takes place when the observer is unable to assign extreme ratings and thus, tends to provide moderate ratings to the observed. The logical error in rating refers to a tendency on the part of the observer to assign similar ratings to the observed for qualities which appear logically related in his own mind (which may not be true otherwise). This type of error differs from halo effect. While in the latter the observer is blindfolded by a favourable (or unfavourable) attitude towards the personality of the observed as a whole, in the former, he is blindfolded by his perceptions as to the relatedness of given qualities regardless of the observed.

MERITS OF RATING SCALE

Notwithstanding the above pitfalls, the effectiveness of the rating scale can be improved using varied measures to overcome them. An attempt may be made to use highly trained multiple observers and pool their ratings. Indeed, in situations where the researcher is interested in larger number of factors, rating scales are more efficient systems. Rating scale systems which contain a wide variety of behaviours at each point on the scale, can provide more data per observer and more dimensions per unit of time. The observer may observe different activities throughout the group meeting, integrate them in his mind and subsequently determine which of the points on a number of scales best represent his interpretation of the varied behaviour. Rating scales are particularly useful in the exploratory or pilot stages in a research study. These scales can also be utilized to summarize and integrate data collected by separate tallies on a category system. This is frequency required to provide a pattern in the data which simple frequency counts on separate observation categories fail to accomplish. Under ideal conditions (which are difficult to achieve), rating can provide data which are comparable to those collected by using a category system of observation. However, if the researcher has adequate resources and requires precision, he is less likely to use rating scales.

REFLECT YOURSELF

1. What are the different types of rating scales?
2. What are the different merits and demerits of rating scales?

INDEX

E

F

G

H

I

J

K

L

M

N